CW00406909

Gareth Jenkins
Precision Attachments
A Link to Successful Restorative Treatment

Precision Attachments
A Link to Successful Restorative Treatment

Gareth Jenkins

BDS FDS RCS MScD
Specialist in Restorative Dentistry
Private Practice in Cardiff, Wales, UK

Technical Contribution by
John Gidden FBIST

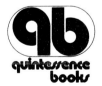

Quintessence Publishing Co Ltd
London, Chicago, Berlin, Tokyo, Paris, Barcelona,
São Paulo, Moscow, Prague and Warsaw

British Library Cataloging in Publication Data
Jenkins, Gareth
Precision attachments : a link to successful restorative treatment
   1. Denture attachments
   1 Title
   617.6'92

ISBN 1850970386

© 1999 Quintessence Publishing Co Ltd

All Rights Reserved
This book or any part thereof must not be reproduced by any means
or in any form without the written permission of the publisher.

Printed and bound by Jütte Druck GmbH, Leipzig, Germany
Litho production by JUP-Industrie- und Presseklischee, Berlin, Germany
Typesetting by Alacrity, Banwell Castle, Weston-super-Mare, UK

Contents

Preface

Precision attachments offer considerable advantages in dentistry because of their flexibility. Nevertheless they have in the past been largely ignored by most dental professionals for understandable reasons: notably cost and an inadequate grasp of their application. The last decade has seen the public become better informed than ever before about the treatment options available to them. There is no doubt that we are already seeing the results of this public awareness in a greater demand for complex restorations. The dental surgeon who familiarizes himself with precision attachments will add a new dimension to his treatment options, and thus also broaden his referral base.

An increase in the popularity of implants, due largely to Brånemark's studies, has brought a concomitant increase in the popularity of precision attachments. It has long been established that attachments can be used to overcome problems of alignment and excessive loss of tissue, both of which are recurring problems in implant work. This makes them invaluable tools in the increasingly popular field of restorative dentistry.

Professionally there can be no greater pleasure or inspiration than to experience the satisfaction and gratitude of patients rehabilitated through the use of techniques and skills offered by modern dentistry. Too often the hopes and aspirations of patients, desperate to be helped to achieve better dental health and fitness, are dashed by those in the profession who are unable to come to terms with the demands of modern dentistry. We have a responsibility to ourselves, our profession and our patients to deliver, whenever possible, the highest standard of dental care of which we are capable.

The aim of this book is to arouse the interest of the general dental practitioner in precision attachments and to illustrate their advantages by presenting (in chapters covering particular patient needs) case studies that can be used as references for treatment planning. It is not intended to be a comprehensive guide to designing removable or fixed prostheses: the reader is referred to the standard texts for that information.

Acknowledgements

My interest in precision attachments goes back to my student days. A part time teacher at Cardiff Dental School, Eric Joseph, aroused a lifelong enthusiasm for the subject. I must thank him for this and, more recently, for advice given in the presentation of this textbook.

I am deeply indebted to Professor J.D. Eccles not only for giving me my first opportunity to develop my clinical skills but also for the confidence, support and encouragement he extended during my early professional life, which has proved invaluable.

I have known John Gidden for many years. His enormous enthusiasm for precision attachments helped develop and sustain my own interest in the subject. He has contributed greatly to my knowledge and for this I will always be grateful. He has also contributed to the technical content of this text, having been involved in treatment planning in many of the cases.

I must also thank Chris Marson and Brian Coleman for their enormous technical support over the years.

Jean Desebrock has worked extremely hard with the drafts and typesetting of the manuscript. I am also grateful to H.W. Haase, Joyce Ronald and all the staff of Quintessence Publishing who have been involved with the production of this text. I am, however, particularly grateful to John Brooks who first approached me and asked if I would be interested in writing this book.

One person must be singled out for her unremitting support and encouragement throughout my professional life, my wife Audrey. She has spent many hours on the word processor deciphering my barely legible handwriting. Numerous drafts were produced and she has helped with the proofreading. I dedicate this book to Audrey, my three children, Alun, Richard and Catrin, and to my parents.

Introduction

Types of Precision Attachment

Precision attachments consist of two halves, a matrix and a patrix, that form a precise but separable joint. They are used to overcome alignment problems where abutments have differing paths of withdrawal, as connectors in fixed partial denture construction and to retain removable partial dentures and overdentures.

Active or Passive Retention

With an *active attachment* the retention between matrix and patrix can be adjusted: this means that the attachment can be reactivated when wear takes place. This makes it an ideal choice to retain a removable partial denture or an overdenture.

With a *passive attachment*, the retention between the elements cannot be increased or decreased. Passive attachments are used mainly to overcome minor alignment problems of abutment teeth, to support the end of a long removable bounded saddle partial denture retained at the opposite end by an active attachment, or to stress break a fixed-movable cemented prosthesis. They are also used in contingency planning.

Rigid or Resilient Attachments

With the *rigid attachment* no movement is possible between the parts. These attachments are usually used in bounded saddle situations, where the abutment teeth fully support the restoration and attachment: the soft tissues do not give any support.

The *resilient attachment* allows movement to take place between the matrix and patrix when fully seated, thus having a stress-breaking function. The movement is usually that of a hinge and serves to distribute potentially harmful forces away from abutment teeth in the free-end saddle situation, and where there are long edentulous spans.

Alloys

A range of different types of alloys is used in the manufacture of attachments: their melting points are generally between 850°C at the lower end and 1450°C at the top end. The porcelain used in porcelain fused to metal restorations has a maturing temperature in the region of 960°C, which is higher than the lower melting point of the attachments.

If attachments from the lower melting point range are chosen and porcelain fused to metal retainers are used, the porcelain stage must be completed first and the attachments post ceramic soldered to the retainers. The big disadvantage of this procedure is that it precludes a full metalwork try-in. It is extremely important to have such a try-in to check the fit of the retainers, the framework of the removable prostheses and the location of the attachments before proceeding to the next stage, the application of porcelain and the set-up of the removable prostheses.

The best choice would therefore be in the higher melting range when porcelain is to be fused to metal as this enables the clinician to carry out a full metal try-in. The technician can incorporate the high melting point attachments into wax patterns and cast onto them when using precious or semi-precious alloys but not when using the high melting point chrome alloys. When an attachment is used in conjunction with yellow gold alloys or processed into acrylic resin, or post ceramic soldered, then an alloy with a lower melting point can be used.

The choice of melting points is a personal one, but in my opinion high melting point attachments, though slightly more expensive, are preferable to low melting point attachments for the above reasons, and also because when soldering there is little risk of melting the attachment if there is a wide differential between the melting points of the attachment and the solder.

Some attachments are supplied as plastic burn-out patterns which are incorporated in the wax pattern and cast in a metal of choice.

Preplanning

Before finally selecting the attachments to be used, study models should be mounted on an articulator using an accurate occlusal registration. The information thus gained is essential for accurately assessing the interarch height at the site of the attachment. The appropriate attachment can then be selected.

Classification of Precision Attachments

This book does not profess to list all available precision attachments. Readers are advised to obtain catalogues from the various manufacturers listed in the Appendix (see page 137). The two main manufacturers of precision attachments are Cendres & Metaux SA and Metaux Precieux SA Metalor, both of Switzerland. In the author's experience the product ranges of attachments produced by these two manufacturers adequately cover the five main classes of attachment, which are:

· Extracoronal
· Intracoronal
· Auxiliary
· Anchors
· Bars.

The following chapters are an introduction to the various types of attachment the author has used over many years and which are described in the Appendix.

1 Treatment Planning

Treatment planning is an essential component of all treatments provided and, unless given the necessary commitment, will result in either failure or relative failure of the case. Essential information which must be obtained to draw up an adequate treatment plan includes:

- Medical and dental history
- Discussion of patient expectations
- Extraoral examination
- Intraoral examination
- Periodontal survey
- Occlusal analysis
- Radiographs
- Study models

Medical and Dental History

The patient's medical and dental history will reveal any obvious problems that could present difficulties either before, during or following any restorative procedures.

Any previous dental history should be recorded carefully and, if the patient has already undertaken restorative work of a complex nature that has failed, then the reasons for such failure must be examined. There may be several reasons, rather than one in particular. An insight into the future success or failure of the proposed reconstruction can sometimes be gained by such investigation. It could well be that, if the fault lay with the patient, unless an improvement can be brought about in the patient's attitude and approach, he or she would be better served with a less complex restorative procedure. However, it should also be recognized that a large proportion of complex failures are not due to the patient's neglect, but rather to the over enthusiasm of a practitioner largely untrained and inexperienced in this field.

The ability of the patient to withstand long clinical procedures should be assessed at this early stage. I have always followed the rule: 'If in doubt do not proceed.' The only exception might be where the patient has little or no alternative to an advanced restorative procedure in order to attain an acceptable level of dental health. In such cases the treatment plan should be as uncomplicated as possible and each appointment short so that all procedures are kept within tolerable limits.

Discussion of Patient Expectations

The value of esthetics is increasingly recognized in modern society. It is at this early stage of planning that patients should be encouraged to comment on the appearance of their existing teeth, and to discuss their desires for the new ones.

Some of them will have a mental picture of what they want; they may even have photographs to show what they have in mind. Older patients will sometimes bring photographs of themselves when they were younger: these are always the most difficult to satisfy and careful counselling may be necessary to achieve an acceptable compromise.

Above all, it is important that patients' hopes are not unrealistically raised by an exaggerated assessment of what can be achieved for them. The truth is kindest in the long run, but it is up to us, as members of a caring profession, to present this as sympathetically as possible, with consideration for patients' feelings.

It must be said that in most cases the results more than satisfy patients' expectations and make this part of our work gratifying and rewarding.

Extraoral Examination

An appraisal can be made almost before the patient is seated in the dental chair. The pallor or healthy glow of the skin, the general state of well-being, can be assessed right at the beginning.

Any asymmetry should be noted, as well as any swellings in the submandibular and sublingual areas. The temporomandibular joint (TMJ) and associated musculature should be examined for any tenderness or pain, as well as for limitation of movement or deviation on opening. Crepitus within the joint itself should also be investigated.

Intraoral Examination

This must include a meticulous examination of all soft tissues, the shape of the ridges and the amount of bone loss. Where gross bone loss precludes the use of conventional fixed partial dentures, precision attachments can often overcome the problem (see Chapters 3 and 4).

The teeth should be examined for caries, the extent of restorations, color, vitality, angulation, mobility and bony support. Tenderness to percussion should be noted as this might indicate periodontal or apical pathology.

Crown lengthening may be necessary for esthetic reasons or for purposes of retention. The length of clinical crowns should be noted. Where a potential abutment tooth has a short clinical crown, electrosurgery should be considered to increase the length of crown sufficiently for the provision of a fixed partial denture or precision attachment. The clinician must, however, consider the biologic width when carrying out such a procedure.[1,2]

Where the gingival contour is uneven, again electrosurgery can be used to improve esthetics.

Periodontal Survey

A full periodontal survey should be carried out. Pocket depths need to be recorded on a periodontal chart and bleeding points noted. The WHO probe is excellent in this respect.

Adequate bony support is essential for fixed prostheses, as well as for any removable prostheses. Full-mouth radiographs taken at the initial visit will determine the level of alveolar bone, the presence of infrabony pockets, the width of the periodontal space and any other anomalies that might exist.

Periodontal disease must be dealt with before carrying out restorative procedures. It is also important that the health of supporting structures is easily maintained following any restorative work carried out for the patient.

Occlusal Analysis

This essential part of all examinations carried out on patients assumes even greater importance when we are dealing with advanced restorative cases requiring major reconstruction.

The dental surgeon should satisfy himself that there are no occlusal interferences that are a cause of existing problems, or could lead to problems at some later stage.

The basic principles of occlusion should be applied to the analysis of each case. These are:

1. There should be a stable co-ordinated occlusal contact of the maximum number of teeth with the mandible in centric relation to the maxilla.
2. There should be a stable co-ordinated occlusal contact with the maximum number of teeth in centric occlusal relationship.
3. Forces should ideally be in line with the long axis of each tooth.
4. There should be no non-working incline contacts.
5. There must be a balance of anterior and posterior inclines.

Premature contacts can, in some cases, lead to parafunctional activity such as bruxism and clenching. The clinician should always look for signs and symptoms, such as excessive wear, TMJ pain, hypersensitivity, hypermobility and fracture lines in teeth.

In cases where there is a considerable derangement of the occlusion due to tooth loss and excessive wear over many years, there may be a need to provide patients with bite-raising appliances, and also with laboratory-made provisional heat-cured acrylic restorations. These can be worn for several months and are invaluable to the clinician in determining the correct vertical dimension and centric relation.

Radiographs

Radiographs are essential for assessing the suitability of teeth and their supporting structures for abutments and the retainers of precision attachments. They will reveal the presence of caries, apical pathology, the condition of the roots, the presence of root fillings and posts, past apisectomies and the architecture and quality of the patient's bone. Orthopantomograph (OPG) radiographs provide an overall view and intraorals are necessary for finer detail. They should be of a suitable standard for accurate diagnosis and for any subsequent medico-legal purposes.

Study Models

Mount these on a semiadjustable articulator using a face-bow and centric record. It will then be possible to assess jaw movements and to examine such items as unit spacing, diastemas and the tilting and overeruption of teeth.

This is the stage at which orthodontics should be considered as part of the treatment plan. Where anterior teeth are missing a wax try-in can be constructed to assess esthetics and to determine whether there is any need to replace lost bone (see Fig 3.7, page 23).

Presentation of the Treatment Plan

It is important that the patient understands his or her problem and its possible solution. The mounted study models and radiographs will help in this. Terminology should be kept simple and easy to understand. The patient should be given time to arrive at a decision: duplicate study models can be taken home for discussion with family or friends. Emphasis should now be laid on the need for correct oral hygiene procedures and regular maintenance of the completed restoration.

A typewritten description of the plan, together with an estimate of the fee, should be presented at this stage and methods of payment indicated. A suitably trained member of staff can deal with this. A professional approach will be appreciated by the patient and will lead to confidence in the dental surgeon and his team.

Case Studies

The following cases illustrate the points made in the previous paragraphs.

Case 1

Figures 1.1 and 1.2 show a case where the patient was wearing a maxillary chrome-cobalt partial denture. The upper left canine and the mandibular incisors had extremely short clinical crowns. These were lengthened using electrosurgery, thus providing sufficient retention for the oral rehabilitation (Fig 1.3). Electrosurgery should be used with a filtered and fully rectified current which allows accurate removal of tissue while causing minimal surrounding damage. The electrode should move quickly, accurately

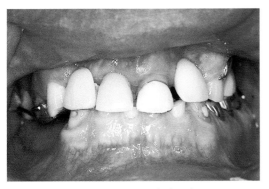

Fig 1.1 Preoperative view with the denture in situ.

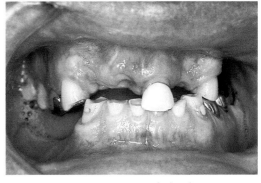

Fig 1.2 Preoperative view with the denture removed, showing excessive wear of the mandibular teeth and the maxillary left canine.

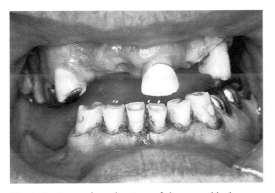

Fig 1.3 Crown lengthening of the mandibular incisors and maxillary left canine using electrosurgery.

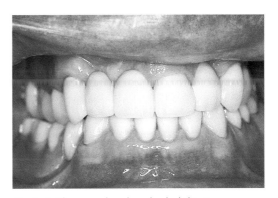

Fig 1.4 The completed oral rehabilitation.

and continuously to achieve the best results. Figure 1.4. shows the finished rehabilitation with precision attachment-retained maxillary and mandibular dentures in both the maxillary left and mandibular right quadrants.

Case 2

Figures 1.5 and 1.6 show a patient with overclosure due to loss of posterior support. Figures 1.7 and 1.8 show the accurately fitting acrylic temporary crowns on which final adjustments were carried out over a three-month period, prior to completion of the case.

Case 3

Figures 1.9 to 1.11 show a directly canti-levered cemented prosthesis replacing a canine which later erupted palatally. It appears that the operator had not taken radiographs.

17

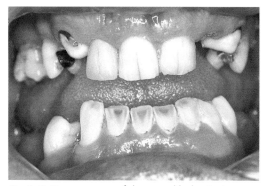

Fig 1.5 Severe wear of the mandibular incisors and canines.

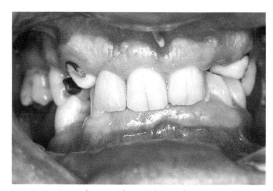

Fig 1.6 Overclosure due to loss of contact following the removal of most of the posterior teeth.

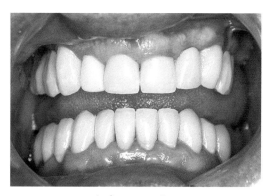

Fig 1.7 Accurately fitting acrylic temporary crowns were adjusted occlusally over a three-month period.

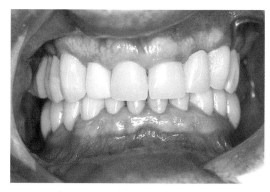

Fig 1.8 The correct centric occlusion was finally re-established at the correct vertical dimension.

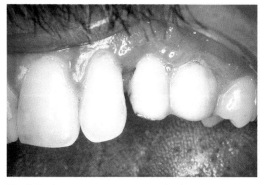

Fig 1.9 An erupting canine pushed a direct cantilever fixed partial denture out of the arch.

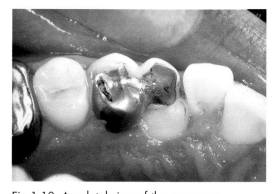

Fig 1.10 A palatal view of the same case.

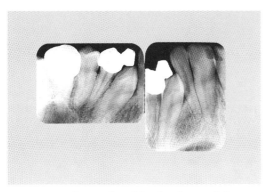

Fig 1.11 Radiographs of the fixed partial denture and canine.

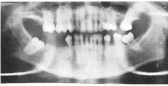
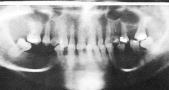
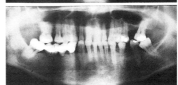

Fig 1.12 Radiograph showing an unerupted mandibular right wisdom tooth before surgical exposure, after eruption and, finally, following fixed partial denture construction.

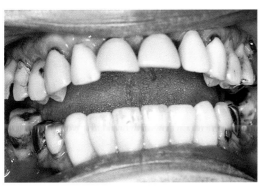

Fig 1.13 The splayed maxillary anterior teeth have lost contact with each other and the lower teeth.

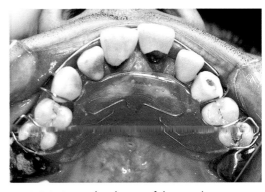

Fig 1.14 An occlusal view of the simple orthodontic appliance used to retract the incisors.

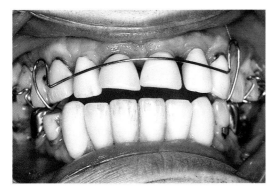

Fig 1.15 A labial view showing loss of the incisal contact.

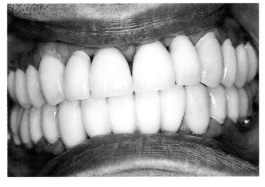

Fig 1.16 The completed work: interproximal contact points, and contact between the maxillary and mandibular incisors, has been re-established.

Case 4

Figure 1.12 shows a case where a 28-year-old woman attended the surgery complaining of a lack of function on the right-hand side of her mouth. Routine radiographs showed that there was an unerupted third molar. This tooth was exposed surgically and the bone over-lying the mesial edge of the crown was removed. The tooth then erupted spontaneously and was left in occlusion for twelve months before being used as an abutment for a fixed partial denture. This allowed reorientation of the fibers of the periodontal ligament for load bearing.

Case 5

Figures 1.13 to 1.16 demonstrate the use of orthodontics to reduce an overjet as well as the anterior open bite, making it possible for the patient to achieve incisal guidance. The treatment also resulted in a marked improvement in appearance.

References

1 *Guargiulo A; Wentz F; Orban B.* Dimensions and relation of the dento-gingival junction. J Periodontal 32: 261-267, 1961.

2 *Kois JC.* Altering gingival levels. The restor-ative connection. Part 1: Biologic variables. J Esthet Dent 6(1): 3-9, 1994.

2 The Free-End Saddle

Precision attachments can transform patients' attitudes to the wearing of removable prostheses. They are more stable and retentive than conventional dentures and for these reasons are better tolerated.

All the basic principles applied to the construction of a good conventional prosthesis should also be applied to the construction of a precision attachment-retained prosthesis. The denture base must cover the maximum area of mucosa of the denture-bearing area as this will provide support and stability. The mandibular free-end saddle denture, unlike the maxillary, has a limited amount of mucosal coverage and, as this is compressible, will result in movement of the prosthesis when under load. The degree of loading and compression of tissue will depend on whether a denture or natural teeth oppose the prosthesis. It will also depend on the muscular development of the patient and the width of the occlusal table.

The denture saddle will depress under occlusal loading until there is a balance between the displacing and resistant forces. It is advisable to take an impression of the mucosa when this is under slight load: for this purpose the author chooses to use a close-fitting acrylic resin tray, fully extended, with a zinc oxide wash. This can be done at the metal try-in stage (when the metal framework is tried in, together with the precision attachment of choice). Having first confirmed that localization of the attachment is correct, the zinc oxide wash can be taken.

Although intracoronal attachments can be used in free-end saddle situations, the author prefers to use extra-coronal attachments. These allow a hinge movement and do not require the preparation of boxes in the distal abutments which may compromise the health of the pulp; extracoronal attachments also obviate the risk of overcontour of the distal portion of the crown, which can result in the accumulation of plaque, gingivitis, pocket formation and carious breakdown in the cervical area.

The same complications are less likely to arise when using extracoronal attachments. These, however, can be positioned too close to the crest of the gingival papilla, a complication seen

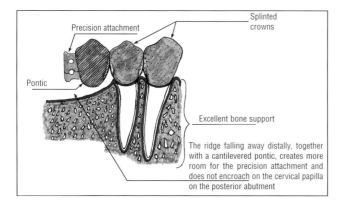

Fig 2.1 and Fig 2.2 Precision attachments connected distally to pontics cantilevered distally were brought more in line with the ridges, reducing the potential for torque on the abutments.

Figure 2.1

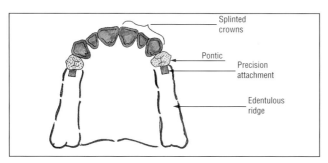

Figure 2.2

when attachments used are too large for the height of clinical crown.

In these circumstances the Mini-Dalbo attachment described in the Appendix (see page 128) can be used without encroachment on the gingival papilla. Alternatively, cantilevering a pontic distally (Fig 2.1) will provide the necessary room for positioning an attachment, by virtue of the increased height available due to the bone loss that occurs distally to the last abutment. It also brings the attachment more in line with the ridges on either side, therefore reducing the potential for torque on the abutment teeth (Fig 2.2).

Bilateral Free-End Saddle Dentures

No one attachment can be used in all situations. The height of the clinical crown is the vital consideration: it must be accurately assessed before the final choice is made. Study models mounted on an articulator enable the distance between the ridge, adjacent to the abutment tooth and the occlusal surface of the opposing arch, to be measured accurately.

Where this height is less than ideal it can, in some circumstances, be increased by surgical means. This is possible only when there is a good thickness of tissue at the proposed attachment site.

Occasionally, teeth in the opposing arch overerupt. It is advisable to deal with this by selective grinding, by crowning where overeruption is greater, or by extraction when it is excessive.

Mounted study models should be correlated against the information obtained from the examination and from radiographs. One can then select the proposed abutment teeth and assess their bony support and the retention which can be expected from their crowns, and also judge their relative paths of withdrawal. After this the clinician and technician will have all the information necessary for selecting the correct attachment.

In cases where the restoration will be opposed by a denture, one tooth only on each side of the arch will be needed as a retainer. Where natural teeth oppose it is usual to include two joined retainers on each side. Needless to say each pair must be parallel and the individual preparations must be sufficiently retentive to prevent one from 'springing off' with disastrous consequences.

Where bony support of the abutment teeth is compromised it may be necessary to include three or more abutment teeth on each side in the design.

Stages in Construction

Case 1

The case shown in Fig 2.3 was a mandibular bilateral free-end saddle opposed by a full maxillary denture. Because of bone loss around the proposed abutment teeth it was

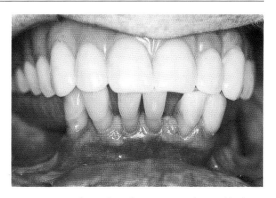

Fig 2.3 Misaligned and unprepared mandibular anterior teeth with bilateral free-end saddles opposing a full maxillary denture.

considered necessary to splint the mandibular lateral incisors and canines on both sides and to use hinging attachments to reduce the stresses upon these abutment teeth.

The attachment of choice was the PR, one to be incorporated on each side distal to the canines. The author has found them to be robust and reliable over many years, with little wear taking place between the patrix and matrix. They are easily reactivated and the complete retention mechanism can be changed in a few moments when it needs renewing.

Stage 1

The six anterior teeth in the mandibular arch were prepared for crowns. An accurate elastomeric impression was taken in a customized tray which had been made from the study model. Temporary crowns were fitted. The impression was poured in artificial stone in the laboratory and accurately fitting heat-cured temporary acrylic crowns were constructed.

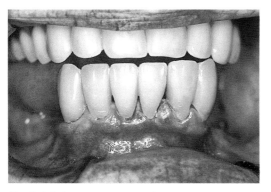

Fig 2.4 Laboratory prepared temporary crowns were fitted. These had been splinted.

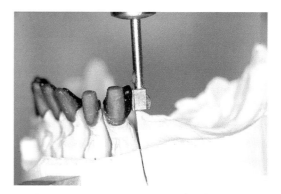

Fig 2.5 Wax patterns were completed on a mandibular model placed on a surveyor. A PR attachment was held in a mandrel with wax built out to contact the attachment.

Stage 2

The laboratory-made temporary crowns were tried in the mouth and assessed for accuracy of fit and occlusion. The final impression of the prepared teeth and the whole denture bearing area was then taken in an elastomeric material, and the laboratory-made temporary crowns temporarily cemented (Fig 2.4).

Stage 3

The final impression was poured using a stone die material. The removable dies were trimmed fully to expose the margins and then painted with model hardener and spaced with die relief, as for conventional crowns and fixed partial denture construction. The model was then placed on a parallelometer (or a surveyor) and the path of insertion determined. This is usually at right angles to the occlusal plane.

After completing the wax patterns, the dies were replaced in the model, which was returned to the parallelometer for alignment of the attachments.

Each attachment has a specific mandril with which it can accurately be oriented to the wax pattern and, ultimately, to the metalwork if soldered (Fig 2.5).

Depending on the type of metal used, many attachments can be incorporated in the wax pattern and have the molten metal cast onto them (see Appendix). Alternatively, the metalwork can be cast without the attachment being present. After casting is completed, the attachment is held in the mandril on the parallelometer, aligned to the casting, secured with sticky wax, invested and soldered.

The author prefers to solder the attachment. If any malalignment has taken place, such as tooth movement, the attachment can readily be removed by heating the metalwork until the solder melts. In this way the attachment, when touched, will fall away. The PR patrix is one example of an attachment made in a high-fusing gold alloy that allows it to be cast onto if required.

Stage 4

When completed, the castings were seated on the master model and placed back on the parallelometer. The PR patrix was then placed in the mandril of the parallelometer and the attachments aligned. Sticky wax was used to secure them to the castings (Fig 2.6). To ensure smooth function of the resilient joints the attachments should, if possible, be parallel in all dimensions (that is, vertically, horizontally and sagittally). If two resilient attachments are used, the axis of rotation should ideally be the same.

Prior to investing, the undersurface of the joint between casting and attachment was relieved with wax for 2 mm on each side to prevent the soldering investment from contacting the casting and the attachment. This enables the solder to flow completely between the two surfaces.

The castings and attachment were then embedded in the soldering investment, with the investment protecting the margins of the castings and the outer surface of the attachment (Fig 2.7). After the investment had set, the wax was boiled away and the area to be soldered was fluxed. The solder used has a melting point of 1060°C.

When soldering was complete, the castings were divested and the oxide on the castings removed by sand blasting with alumina grit. It is important that the attachments are not sandblasted, but cleaned using a glass fiber brush. The castings were then placed back on the model (Fig 2.8).

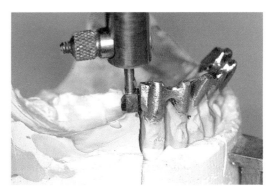

Fig 2.6 The attachments were aligned on the surveyor and sticky waxed to the finished castings.

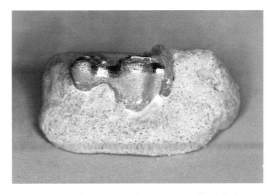

Fig 2.7 Attachments and castings embedded in soldering investment.

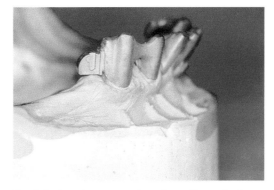

Fig 2.8 Attachments and castings divested, air abraded and replaced on the working model.

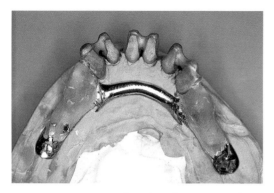

Fig 2.9 A PR matrix placed on the patrix and localized to the chrome-cobalt lingual bar with autopolymer resin.

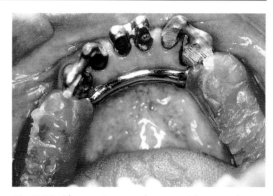

Fig 2.10 The castings and removable partial denture were tried in the mouth. Centric occlusion can be checked again at this stage.

Stage 5

A chrome-cobalt lingual bar connector was cast and finished, placed on the fixed model, and secured in position with sticky wax. The patrix was placed in the matrix, with care being taken to ensure that it was fully seated. The undersurface of the attachment and the ridge on which it rested was blocked out with wax to prevent the autopolymer resin, used to localize the attachment to the chrome-cobalt lingual bar, from running under the matrix, preventing separation of the removable partial denture and the castings. Autopolymer resin was used to localize the matrix to the lingual bar (Fig 2.9).

Stage 6

A complete trial of the metal components was then carried out in the patient's mouth in order to check the accuracy of the previous stages.

The fit of the "fixed" component was first checked; then the removable section

was gently inserted. This should seat down fully without causing discomfort to the patient and without displacing the "fixed" section (Fig 2.10). This was first carried out with the attachments deactivated and then with them activated so that one could feel and hear the click as they engaged fully.

Provided temporization is good no problems should arise at this stage. Any movement of the "fixed" section would probably be due to tooth movement and subsequent misalignment of the patrices.

Some operators carry out the above stage with the porcelain crowns completed so that they can be checked for esthetics and occlusion. Those who are unfamiliar with this type of work should defer this to a separate stage since the completed porcelain makes it more difficult to detect inaccuracies.

Centric occlusion should be checked at this stage using 'check back' techniques, and re-recorded if necessary (Fig 2.10).

Final Stages

These correspond to the routine stages of denture construction. The denture teeth are set up on the articulated master model and tried in the mouth for fit and occlusion (Fig 2.11).

It is important to block out the matrices with plaster before processing the acrylic in order to prevent it from flowing into them.

The denture is processed on a duplicate model, an acrylic base or a model made from an accurately adapted wax base. When completed it is returned to the master model to check accuracy and, if necessary, to adjust the occlusion by grinding.

Figure 2.12 shows the completed case on the model and Figs 2.13 to 2.15 the completed case fitted in the mouth.

Unilateral Free-End Saddles

Unilateral free-end saddles can be used in an otherwise intact arch, or in combination with a bounded saddle on the opposite side of the arch.

Case 2

Figure 2.16 shows a typical example of a unilateral free-end saddle on the right side in combination with a bounded saddle which, in this case, spans 11 to 16.

Teeth present were 6,8,9,10,11 and 16. It was decided to splint the left lateral incisor and canine and bridge the space between the maxillary right central incisor and the canine. PR attachments were then used as extracoronal attachments, connected distally to both

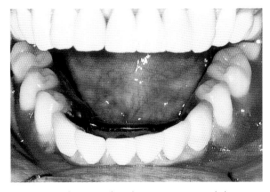

Fig 2.11 The completed restorations and the precision attachment denture were tried in the mouth and checked for fit and centric occlusion. At this stage the teeth on the denture were set up in wax.

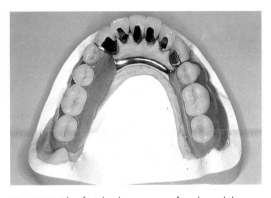

Fig 2.12 The finished case on a fixed model.

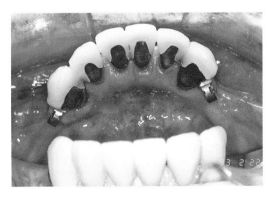

Fig 2.13 The crowns fitted and following a better alignment than in Fig 2.3.

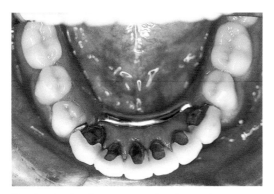

Fig 2.14. The denture seated with good adaptation of the lingual bar.

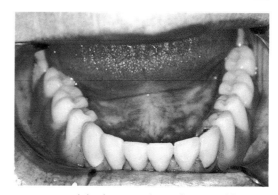

Fig 2.15 A labial view with no clasps visible.

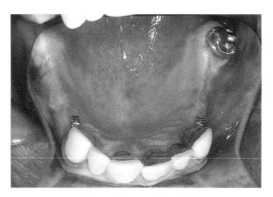

Fig 2.16 A unilateral free-end saddle in combination with a bounded saddle. The crowns at 10 and 11 were splinted and carried a PR attachment off the distal of the canine. On the other side a fixed partial denture replacing 7 also had a PR attachment off the distal of 6.

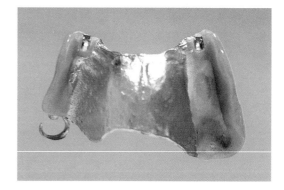

Fig 2.17 The fitting surface of the denture with the matrices of the PR attachments processed in acrylic.

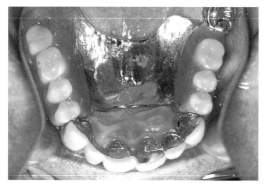

Fig 2.18 The prosthesis fitted.

canines. Additional support and cross-arch stabilization were provided by using a chrome-cobalt palate to connect the saddles (Figs 2.17 and 2.18).

Patients should be told, when presented with their treatment plans, of the importance of correct oral hygiene procedures, and should understand that they will need to return regularly so that the reconstruction can be checked and any necessary corrections made. It is particularly important to compensate for bone resorption by rebasing the saddle areas, as gross resorption can throw undue stresses upon the abutment teeth.

The case shown was completed more than twenty-five years ago when acrylic-faced gold crowns were in common use.

Case 3

Precision attachments provide the ideal solution to the problem of the unilateral free-end saddle (Figs 2.19 to 2.21). Since there could be considerable torque on the prosthesis from opposing natural teeth, a robust attachment such as the PR should be used with two or more abutment teeth providing retention and resistance to torque. It is an advantage if the shape of the bony ridge also provides resistance to lateral forces and such favorable anatomy obviates the need for cross-arch stabilization. Patients appreciate the comfort of such a simple design.

Teeth present in this case were 6, 8, 11 and 13 to 16, 22 to 31. There was limited posterior support. The reasons for this were twofold: firstly, the permanent teeth remaining in the mandibular right quadrant were opposed by a maxillary partial chrome-cobalt denture and, secondly, the permanent teeth remaining in the maxillary left quadrant were not in occlusion, as the patient had not been wearing a mandibular partial denture.

Solid posterior support, as where natural teeth with wide occlusal tables oppose each other, did not exist. This placed considerable stress on the anterior teeth and had, apparently, caused the earlier loss of two anterior teeth due to root fracture. Both had previously been restored by post crowns.

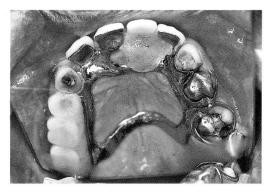

Fig 2.19 The maxillary arch prior to treatment.

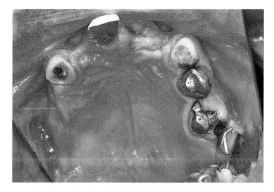

Fig 2.20 A unilateral free-end saddle and standing teeth heavily restored.

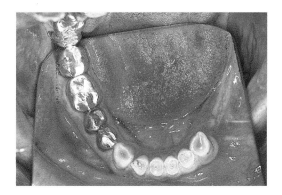

Fig 2.21 Severely attrited mandibular incisors and canines with a unilateral free-end saddle distal to the mandibular left canine.

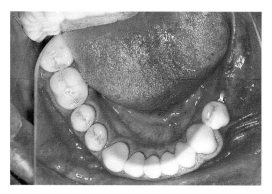

Fig 2.22 Mandibular crowns fitted, with 22 to 24 splinted and a cantilevered pontic at 21 with a PR attachment distally placed.

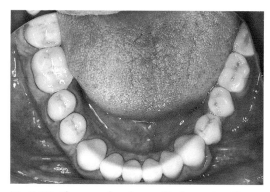

Fig 2.23 The completed mandibular arch with a removable unilateral denture in position. Note that there is no lingual bar or clasping.

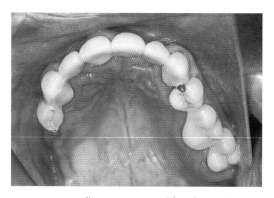

Fig 2.24 Maxillary crowns and fixed partial dentures fitted with a PR attachment connected distally to the 5 pontic.

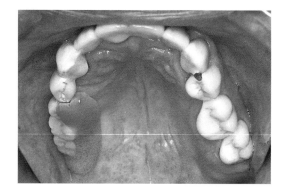

Fig 2.25 The completed maxillary arch with the removable denture in place. There was little coverage of the palate.

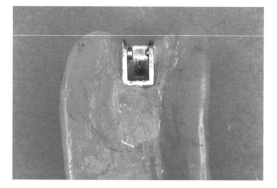

Fig 2.26 The fitting surface of the unilateral denture with the matrix processed in acrylic.

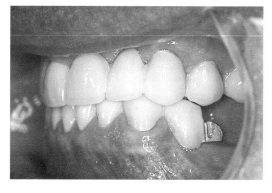

Fig 2.27 The cantilevered pontic 21 allowed more interarch height for the attachment.

Some solid posterior support in the maxillary right quadrant was achieved by cantilevering a pontic in the first premolar position from the splinted central and lateral incisors and canine. A pontic was similarly cantilevered in the mandibular left first premolar position. Each pontic carried a PR attachment retaining a unilateral prosthesis.

Figures 2.22 and 2.23 show the completed mandibular arch with 21 pontic and PR attachment, Figs 2.24 and 2.25 the maxillary arch with 5 pontic and PR attachment, and Fig 2.26 the fitting surface of the maxillary prosthesis.

Cantilevered pontics carrying attachments can solve a number of problems. They can improve esthetics in the anterior part of the mouth where it is not desirable to see the bulk of an attachment or the junction of the fixed and removable sections. They enable the unsightly attachment to be moved further back in the arch, eg from a maxillary lateral to a maxillary canine position.

They can also cantilever the axis of rotation to a less curved part of the arch, allowing attachments to be placed parallel, and they can often be used to place attachments in positions where more vertical height is available (Fig 2.27).

Case 4

Figures 2.28 and 2.29 are preoperative views of a free-end saddle distal to the maxillary left lateral incisor. The maxillary central incisors and left lateral incisors were splinted with crowns cantilevering the 11 pontic, which carried an attachment at 12 (Fig 2.30). In such

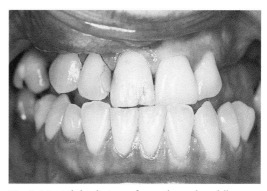

Fig 2.28 A labial view of a unilateral saddle which extended distally to 10. The patient had a Class III jaw relationship.

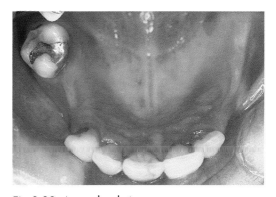

Fig 2.29 An occlusal view.

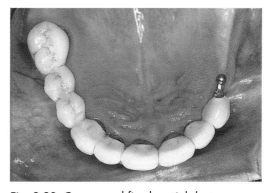

Fig 2.30 Crowns and fixed partial dentures fitted showing a directly cantilevered pontic at 11 with a Dalbo attachment placed distally.

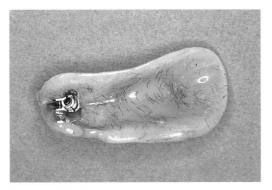

Fig 2.31 The fitting surface of the maxillary denture. Note that the acrylic had been relieved on both sides adjacent to the spring leaf to allow this to be opened or closed depending on the amount of retention required.

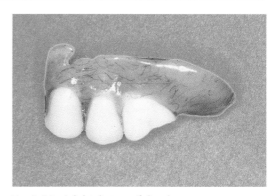

Fig 2.32 A labial view of the denture.

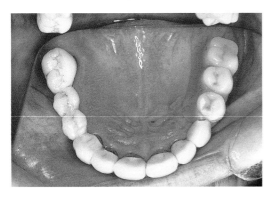

Fig 2.33 The denture viewed occlusally is seen to cover little of the palate.

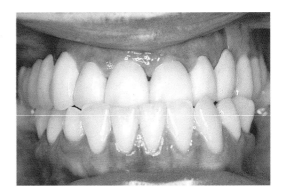

Fig 2.34 A labial view with the teeth in centric occlusion.

a case the connection of 10 and 11 must be large and hence strong enough to carry the cantilever without encroaching upon the distal gingival contour — not possible if the natural teeth had been short.

Figure 2.30 also shows how the cantilever allows the attachment to be placed more favorably in the arch. Figures 2.31 and 2.32 show the removable prosthesis, Fig 2.33 is a mirror image, and Fig 2.34 the completed case.

3 The Bounded Saddle

Bounded saddles can arise in either the anterior or posterior part of the mouth. They can be found in combination with free-end saddles or with other bounded saddles in the same arch. They are generally easier to treat than free-end saddles and provide better treatment options where clinicians are aware of the alternatives available.

Anterior-Bounded Saddles

Problems which might arise in this situation and complicate the provision of conventional fixed partial dentures could be due to:

· bone loss
· unit spacing
· lack of parallelism of abutment teeth and preparations.

Bone Loss

Where bone loss has been only slight and a "gum fitted" fixed partial denture is acceptable in appearance, no problem arises. Small deficiencies can be corrected by adding pink porcelain between the pontics.

Case 1

Figure 3.1 shows how pink porcelain placed between the pontics anteriorly allows a more normal appearance. It avoids unsightly black triangles or the "squaring" of the cervical margins which would result were tooth-colored porcelains not used to close the deficiencies.

Greater loss of bone requires a bone augmentation procedure (prior to fitting either a fixed partial denture or an implant supported prosthesis) or else a removable prosthesis retained by precision attachments. The latter is not only less expensive but also avoids the need for surgery, while fulfilling both functional and esthetic demands. It is often an attractive alternative to patients.

Case 2

Figures 3.2 and 3.3 show the loss of the four maxillary incisors, left canine and right first premolar, with adjacent tissues, due to a road traffic accident. The existing maxillary partial chrome-cobalt denture lacked retention and stability and

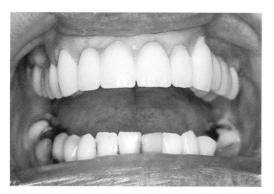

Fig 3.1 Pink porcelain placed cervically in the embrasures of 7, 8 and 8, 9.

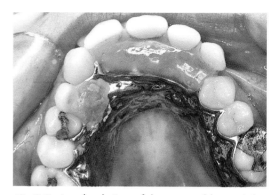

Fig 3.2 A palatal view of the removable partial denture worn.

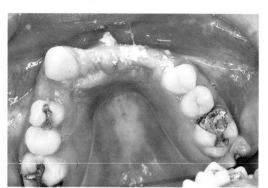

Fig 3.3 Note the position of the anterior teeth in Fig 3.2 in relation to the bone loss shown here. Denture fixative can be seen, which was necessary to retain the denture.

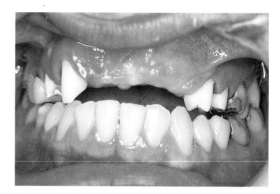

Fig 3.4 The prepared abutment teeth. Clearance for a full coverage of porcelain was provided.

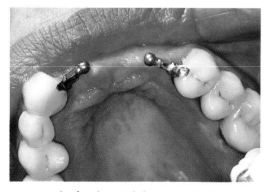

Fig 3.5 The fixed partial denture at 4, 5, 6 and splinted crowns at 12, 13 which carried Mini-Dalbos anteriorly.

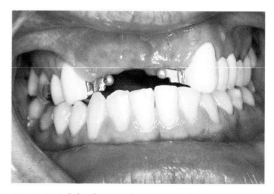

Fig 3.6 A labial view showing the limited space available for the attachments. The attachment on the patient's left side lay lingually to the mandibular canine.

was unacceptable to the patient. Full crowns were used to provide retention when bridging the missing 5. Premolars 12 and 13 were splinted with joined crowns and Mini-Dalbo attachments were soldered to 6 and 12. They are particularly useful in situations where there is restricted vertical height so that other larger attachments are precluded.

Figure 3.4 shows the prepared teeth, and Figs 3.5 and 3.6 the fixed components in the mouth. Figure 3.7 shows the bulk of acrylic that was necessary to replace the missing tissue. Figures 3.8 and 3.9 are views of the completed restoration.

Case 3

In cases where only a small removable flange is necessary the Gaussen attachment can be used to make such a flange for a fixed partial denture. This is a useful procedure where bone loss is not considerable, but where pink porcelain would not suffice.

The case shown in Figs 3.10 and 3.11 illustrates loss of bone in the maxillary incisor region with the added complication of an instanding canine, 6. There was no problem in aligning the 5, 6 and 11 preparations but the crossbite presented risks in using a conventional soldered joint between 6 and 7 pontics. A palatal bar connector was used to overcome the problem.

The matrix of the Gaussen attachment was housed in 8 pontic, and the removable acrylic flange was processed onto the matrix (Fig 3.12). When inserted, a depression in the patrix engaged a spring loaded plunger. The mechanism is replaceable. A single Gaussen will suffice for gumwork involving up to four teeth.

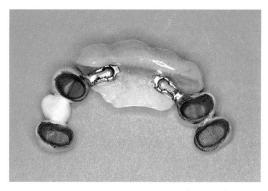

Fig 3.7 The thickness of the labial flange shows the amount of bone loss.

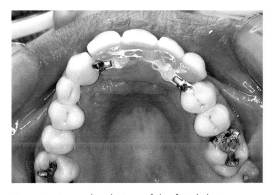

Fig 3.8 An occlusal view of the fitted denture.

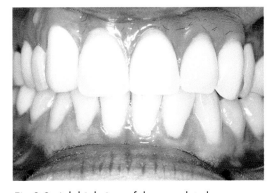

Fig 3.9 A labial view of the completed case.

35

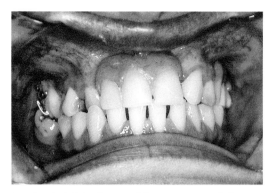

Fig 3.10 A labial view of the conventional denture worn to replace the missing central incisors and maxillary right lateral incisor. Note the crossbite on the right side and the instanding canine.

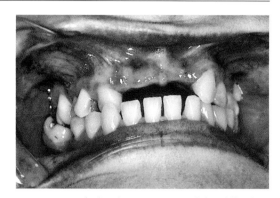

Fig 3.11 With the denture removed the difficulty of the instanding canine can be seen more clearly.

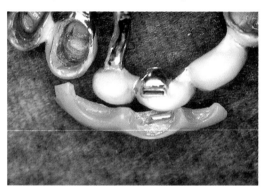

Fig 3.12 A Gaussen PA placed in the pontic of 8 retained a removable acrylic flange.

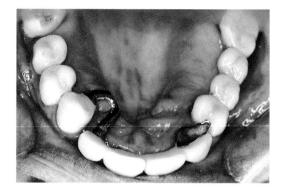

Fig 3.13 A palatal bar connector circumvented the problem of the instanding canine. The 11 crown was connected to the 12 crown by means of an interlock.

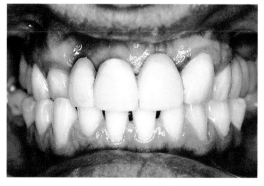

Fig 3.14 A labial view without the acrylic flange in place.

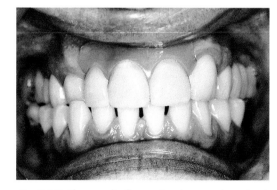

Fig 3.15 The acrylic flange in place and retained by the Gaussen attachment.

Figure 3.13 is a palatal view, and Figs 3.14 and 3.15 labial views, the first without and the second with the flange in position.

Patients should be given instruction in the insertion, removal and cleaning of their appliances.

Unit Spacing

Where all maxillary incisors between the canines are missing and the span is long, due to the presence of diastemas between the lost teeth, the provision of a fixed partial denture may be impractical. An alternative treatment would be the provision of a removable partial denture, using teeth on either side of the space for support and the retention of precision attachments similar to those shown in Fig 3.5.

This situation occurs only rarely. Usually all but the longest anterior spans can be restored by slightly over-contouring the pontics to close the diastemas, or by using a palatal bar connector as shown in Fig 3.13.

Lack of Parallelism of Abutment Teeth and Preparations

When proposed abutment teeth on either side of an anterior-bounded saddle have divergent angles which prevent crown preparations from being parallel, conventional fixed partial dentures are not possible. Where proposed abutment teeth on one side of the saddle can be made parallel, but not to those of the other side, the

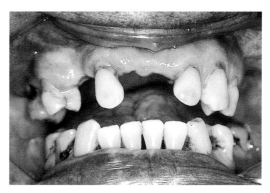

Fig 3.16 Proclined lateral incisors made alignment with the posterior teeth impossible.

solution is to make a removable partial denture on extracoronal attachments.

A situation might occasionally arise where one abutment on one side of a space anteriorly can be made parallel to one on the other side, but these alone would not provide sufficient support for the missing anterior teeth. Increased support from adjacent teeth with slightly different paths of withdrawal which are not extreme can be provided by using interlocks such as the Stern Tube-lock to connect retainers.

Case 4

The use of this attachment is illustrated in the following case where the patient had lost both maxillary central incisors many years previously and found a partial maxillary denture so uncomfortable that she would not wear it (Fig 3.16). 2, 5, 7, 10, 11 and 12 were present. Both lateral incisors were proclined and could not therefore be included in the proposed posterior fixed partial dentures (Figs 3.17 and 3.18).

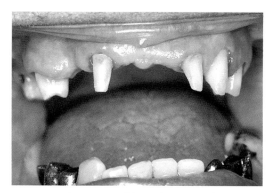

Fig 3.17 The prepared lateral incisors share a path of withdrawal, but not with the posterior teeth.

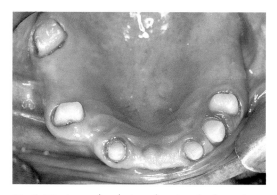

Fig 3.18 An occlusal view showing the lateral incisor proclination.

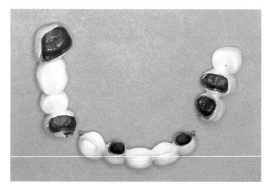

Fig 3.19 The three separate units of the fixed partial dentures completed.

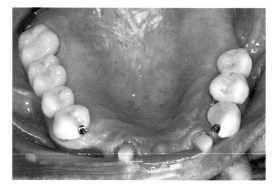

Fig 3.20 Interlocks in the mesial surfaces of the maxillary canine and premolar had the same path of insertion as the anterior fixed partial dentures.

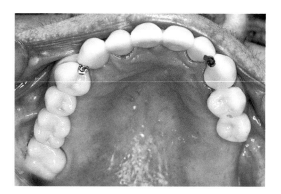

Fig 3.21 An occlusal view showing the three fixed partial dentures connected with interlocks, which greatly increased support to the anterior fixed partial denture and solved the problem of the teeth not being aligned.

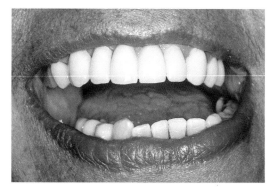

Fig 3.22 A happy patient, previously unable to tolerate a removable partial denture.

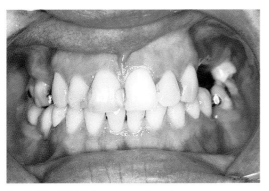

Fig 3.23 A labial preoperative view.

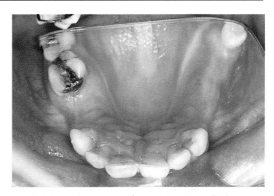

Fig 3.24. A long span from 11 to 16 which was bucally inclined precluded conventional fixed partial dentures. There was also considerable bone loss in the edentulous saddle area.

The problem was solved by using Stern Tube-locks in the distal of 10 crown and 6 pontic to link up with the posterior fixed partial dentures (Figs 3.19 and 3.20). The completed case is shown in Figs 3.21 and 3.22.

Posterior-Bounded Saddles

As with the anterior-bounded saddle, problems involving bone loss and divergent abutment teeth arise. Unit spacing is not such a problem posteriorly as it is in the anterior part of the mouth, and it is usually possible to satisfy the less demanding esthetic requirements by under- or overcontouring the pontics. However it must be emphasized that this should only be slight.

Conventional fixed partial dentures are ruled out when one of the proposed abutment teeth is compromised by poor bony support or an undersized root.

The same applies to a very long pontic span. Precision attachments provide the solution to these problems.

Case 5

Figures 3.23 and 3.24 show a span from 11 to 16. The latter was not only a small tooth but also had a buccal inclination. There had been considerable bone loss along the length of the saddle. All these factors contraindicated fixed partial dentures.

The splinted crowns on the maxillary left lateral incisor and canine were used to carry a Mini-Dalbo precision attachment on the distal of 11 and the removable section was further secured by a Stern Tube-lock in the crown on 16. Needless to say, these two attachments had to be paralleled on the master model.

Figure 3.25 shows the fixed components in the mouth and Fig 3.26 the removable section. The spring leaves of

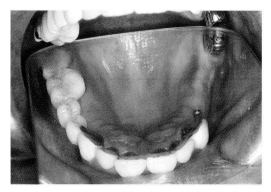

Fig 3.25 A crown and fixed partial denture fitted with a Mini-Dalbo attachment off the distal of 11, and a full gold crown on 16 with an interlock mesially aligned to the Mini-Dalbo.

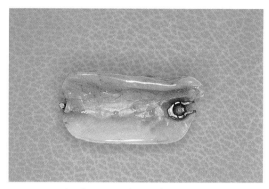

Fig 3.26 The fitting surface of the acrylic denture into which the two attachments were processed. The technician had been careful to relieve the acrylic adjacent to the spring leaves.

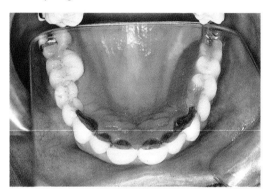

Fig 3.27 An occlusal view of the completed case.

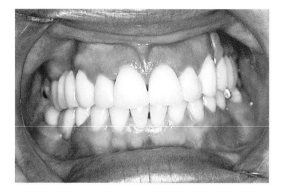

Fig 3.28 A labial view of the completed case.

the matrix must be allowed to move outwards as they pass over the ball of the patrix. The technician will have relieved the acrylic in this area prior to delivery but the clinician should also check that this relief is adequate. Figures 3.27 and 3.28 show the completed case.

4 Overdentures

When patients present with only a few remaining teeth in their mouths which may show varying degrees of overeruption, tilting and mobility, these should not be extracted before considering the advantages to the patient of retaining their roots and thus the surrounding alveolar bone. These roots can give stability and retention to an overdenture and provide proprioception which would otherwise be lost with a full denture.

The crowns must be resected and the root canals filled. Any periodontal problems will need to be resolved by the usual techniques which will include root planing and possibly periodontal surgery to deal with infra-bony pockets. Once this has been carried out even teeth with grade one mobility can be used providing that patients carry out scrupulous oral hygiene measures around them.

Many patients who are unhappy about the fit of their full dentures will nowadays undergo lengthy procedures at considerable expense involving implants and, sometimes, bone grafting. Healthy retained roots are natural implants and, although some may have a limited length of usefulness, using them will improve the quality of patients' lives.

Anchors or Stud Attachments

Anchors, also known as stud attachments, are made in rigid form for bounded saddle situations and in resilient form for free-end saddles. Since they are relatively simple to use they are a good introduction to precision attachments for the practitioner and technician. They are generally used in conjunction with posts and diaphragms placed in root canals following root canal therapy.

A typical case would be where the patient has a few remaining mandibular anterior teeth which have overerupted, interfering with the occlusion of a full maxillary denture. This situation, where the posterior ridges have become flattened by resorption, is seen frequently in elderly patients.

Wearing a mandibular denture is something that most patients find very difficult, especially as they get older, because neuromuscular control diminishes and with it the ability to adapt

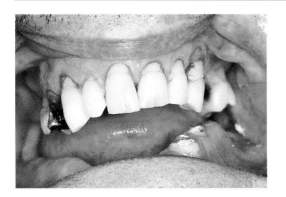

Fig 4.1 The three remaining teeth at 20, 21 and 22 were decoronated. Note the substantial amount of bone available in this area in comparison with the rest of the mandibular arch.

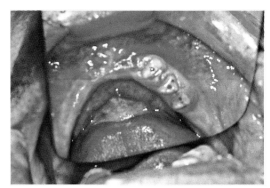

Fig 4.2 After being decoronated the teeth were prepared for posts and diaphragms.

easily to something new in the mouth. More of our patients are now retaining their teeth into late middle and old age and this group presents the greatest prosthetic challenge to the clinician.

It is not uncommon for patients to have lost all but two or three of their teeth. These can nevertheless be retained provided that there has not been too much bone loss and no pathological pockets remain.

Overeruption of these teeth may however reduce the interocclusal space available in which to house the attachment, denture base and teeth. In such circumstances gingivectomy may occasionally enable the height of the root face to be lowered, thus providing more room.

Anchors are usually retained by means of posts with diaphragms. Since they will be subject to considerable displacement forces during removal of the prosthesis, great care must be taken to ensure that they are sufficiently retentive. The author uses a dentin-bonding resin which bonds to the complete dentin surface of the

canal and root face. The metal surfaces are sandblasted and tin-plated to enhance the bond. Important supplementary retention is achieved at the cementation stage by the use of a separate nonparallel pin through the diaphragm into the dentin, provided that there is sufficient bulk of root.

Case 1

The case shown in Figs 4.1 to 4.10 was dealt with by removing the crowns and root filling the mandibular left canine and premolars. The root canals were prepared for posts (Figs 4.1 and 4.2) and the root surfaces reduced as low as possible to accommodate the diaphragms and attachments which were to be placed in the middle of the preparations and above the post hole.

Impressions of the post crown preparations and the denture-bearing area were taken in a stock tray modified with composition to ensure that it was correctly extended. Temporary crowns can be made for each preparation, or an existing

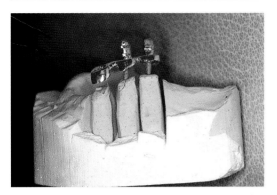

Fig 4.3 Posts and diaphragms were constructed for 20 and 21, and a diaphragm with an aperture and lock only for the canine as this root canal had a different path of withdrawal from the premolar root canals.

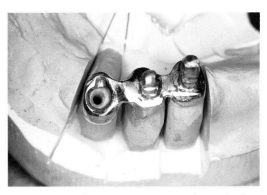

Fig 4.4 Consideration was given to the path of insertion of the post in the canine when designing the wax pattern for the diaphragm incorporating the aperture and lock.

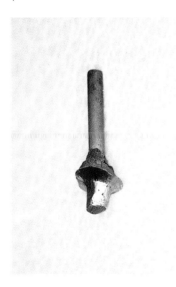

Fig 4.5 The post with its locating core was constructed to fit through the diaphragm for 22.

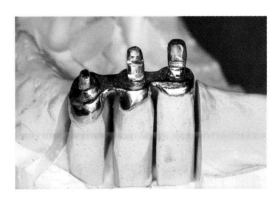

Fig 4.6 Posts and diaphragms with their locating cores ready for the final impression.

denture can be adapted in the laboratory. In this case the patient did not wear a mandibular denture and conventional dressings sufficed.

The technician constructed the posts and diaphragms with locating cores about 10 mm high (Figs 4.3 and 4.4). Since the path of withdrawal of the canine differed from that of the premolars, a separate post was constructed which passed through an aperture in the diaphragm of 22 splinting it to the joined 20, 21 restorations (Figs 4.5 and 4.6). This is an extremely retentive device.

The castings were tried in the mouth for accuracy of fit and for retention (Fig 4.7). When this was achieved, an overall impression of the castings and the saddle

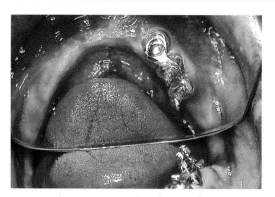

Fig 4.7 The castings tried in the mouth.

areas was taken in a special tray using an accurate impression material. Grooves cut in the locating cores assisted in accurate placing of the posts and diaphragms in the impression.

Where there are no path of withdrawal problems an alternative method would be to cut holes in the special tray over the localizing cores and fix them to the tray with autopolymer resin.

Resilient **Eccentric Rothermann anchors** were used in this case. They are very shallow and easy for the technician to use because they incorporate their own solder. They consist of a clasp arm which is the matrix engaging an undercut on a shallow cylinder which is the patrix. When using two or more anchors they need not be precisely parallel. The diaphragms can be milled parallel and the Eccentric cylinders placed on them.

In order to prevent 20, 21 and 22 from being stressed by the long saddle from 31 to 23 marks on the patrices of the anchors allowed the technician to orient them so that the retentive arms of the

matrices functioned correctly. These marks were transferred to the milled gold diaphragms, thus avoiding errors prior to soldering.

An acrylic base was constructed, keeping the areas around the remaining canine and premolar roots clear. For a resilient prosthesis, a spacer must be used to prevent the fitting surface of the prosthesis from contacting the diaphragm. Two tin spacer discs are provided with each attachment: a large one to burnish over the diaphragm and a small one to sit on top of the patrix.

Since it is not easy to burnish the large tin spacer, the diaphragm can be relieved with sheet wax (0.5 mm thick). The matrices are placed on the patrices, lining up the space between the arms to the mark on the patrices. The small tin spacers are placed on top of the patrices and wax is poured around the outer surfaces of the matrices. This allows some relief between the arms of the matrices and the fitting surface of the prosthesis, ensuring that the arms are kept free to move.

Spacers are not used with the rigid attachment, but it is essential to relieve the arms of the matrices in the same way.

Autopolymer acrylic resin was used to cover and localize the attachments to the acrylic base. When cured, the wax relief was removed, after which the normal stages of denture construction were carried out.

The posts and diaphragms and attachments were seated in position (Fig 4.8). Marginal adaptation was again checked and the overdenture was tried in. There should be positive clicks as the denture seats correctly. When this was confirmed, the occlusion was checked, followed by the esthetic result. The denture was then processed off the master model using the original acrylic base (Fig 4.9).

The final stage was to try in the attachments and denture, to ensure that no errors had been introduced between appointments that would have prevented its correct seating. Once it was certain that the fit was accurate, the whole of the preparation area was made ready and the fixed components were cemented in place.

Excess cement was cleaned off and the denture was seated. There should be no rocking around the attachments and the occlusion should be corrected, either immediately in the mouth or by taking a precentric record and adjusting on the articulator after remounting. There should be audible clicks as the attachments engage.

The patient was given careful instruction on home care with particular attention to plaque control, both around the root diaphragms and attachments, and the fitting surface of the denture. Ideally the dental hygienist should advise the patient in this respect.

Figure 4.10 shows the finished work. The maxillary arch was restored using conventional crowns and a fixed partial denture, as well as a precision attachment-retained unilateral partial denture.

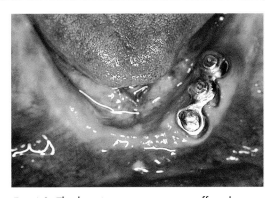

Fig 4.8 The locating cores were cut off and two Eccentric Rothermann anchors were soldered to the premolar diaphragms.

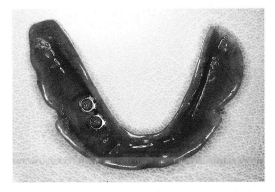

Fig 4.9 The fitting surface of the denture with the matrices processed in acrylic. It is essential that the acrylic adjacent to the arms of the matrices is relieved to allow them to spring over the patrices.

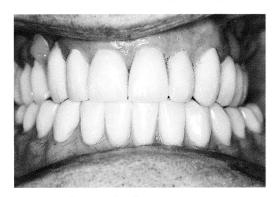

Fig 4.10 The completed case.

Bar Attachments

Spaced teeth which are splinted by a bar are mutually supportive: in the author's experience they last longer than individual teeth. Many bar attachments have been developed over the years. Carr[1] in 1898 was the first to introduce cast alloy bar patterns to dentistry. Early this century Bennett[2] and Fossume[3] used round bar patterns attached to gold crowns to support a removable superstructure. The Dolder bar has been used for more than fifty years. Burn-out resin patterns are available and custom-made bars can be milled in the laboratory.

The **Ackermann bar** is probably the most versatile and popular factory-made model. There are two types of bar: round and egg shaped. One advantage of the round bar is that it can be bent in all directions and can be constructed to follow not only the antero-posterior relationship, but also the vertical changes in the arch. The egg shaped bar has extra rigidity making bending more difficult.

A half-round brass wire (0.7 mm) is used as a spacer and is provided with each clip. This spacer will allow vertical movement. In cases where a straight bar is used between two implants or two teeth, rotational movement will also take place. The precious metal clip is only 3.6 mm in length, which enables it to be used in areas of short span. Retention in the denture is achieved by using tags embedded in the acrylic. There are two designs of clip that allow retention in either a buccolingual direction or along the length of the bar.

The Ackermann bar is available in two different types of metal. The first is a high fusing alloy with a melting point in the range of 1400-1460°C. If this metal is used it can be cast onto or soldered. It is particularly useful if used in conjunction with porcelain fused to metal retainers as it avoids post ceramic soldering.

The other metal is a gold-palladium alloy with a melting range of 935-1065°C. This alloy must be soldered to the castings. Rather than soldering the ends of the bar it is advisable to extend the wax approximately 1.5 mm from the gold cylinder to form a cradle into which the bar will localize. When the patterns are cast and trimmed the bar is localized into the extensions and then sticky waxed in this position. The metalwork is then removed from the model, invested in soldering investment and soldered. A stronger joint between the bar and the castings will be provided in this way: it does not rely on the small area of contact between the ends of the bar and the castings.

Case 2

A situation which commonly arises, a patient who has just two mandibular canines remaining from the original dentition, is shown in Figs 4.11 to 4.13. This case had previously been restored by his former dentist with gold copings and a simple overdenture but the patient was not satisfied with its stability and retention.

A decision was taken to remove the existing copings and replace them with two new ones, at the same time

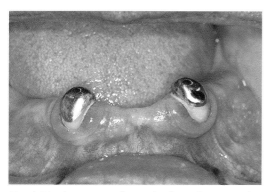

Fig 4.11 A previous dentist had wisely retained the roots of the two mandibular canines, placing gold copings on them.

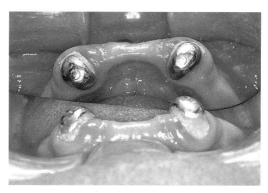

Fig 4.12 An occlusal view shows that the canines were ideally positioned for the construction of a bar.

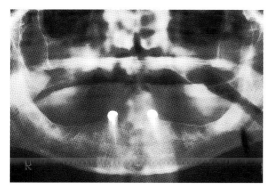

Fig 4.13 A radiograph showed good length of roots well supported by bone.

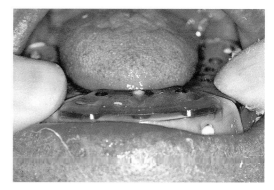

Fig 4.14 An alginate impression was taken over the existing gold copings at the commencement of treatment.

utilizing the maximum length of root possible above the apical seal of the root fillings. Before removing the copings an alginate impression was taken for construction of the temporary copings (Fig 4.14).

The gold copings were then removed (Fig 4.15) and the root canals prepared for posts of maximum length. Para posts were placed in each root canal and an impression was taken (Figs 4.16 and 4.17).

Temporary copings made from the alginate impression taken at the commencement of treatment were fixed to Dentatus screws in the root canals (Figs 4.18 and 4.19). Having cast the model the technician waxed up and cast the posts and diaphragms and joined them with an Ackermann bar (Fig 4.20).

The technician constructed a special tray fitting over the copings and bar and extended to cover the full denture-bearing area. The metalwork was then

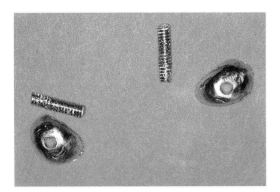

Fig 4.15 The gold posts and copings were removed.

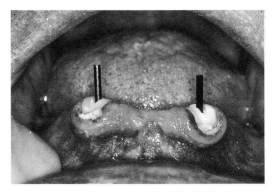

Fig 4.16 Para posts were placed in both canines, and retraction cord in the gingival crevice of each tooth. An overall impression was taken.

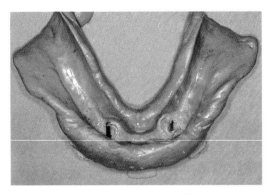

Fig 4.17 The overall impression before the working model was poured.

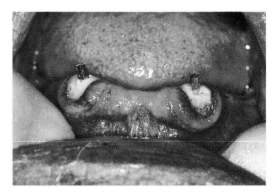

Fig 4.18 Dentatus screws in both canals helped to retain the temporary copings constructed from the alginate impression taken at the commencement of treatment.

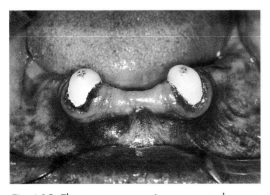

Fig 4.19 The temporary copings cemented.

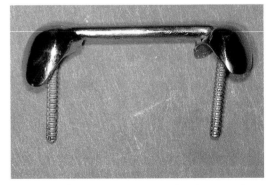

Fig 4.20 The posts, copings and Ackermann bar. Note the length of the posts.

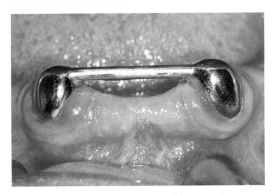

Fig 4.21 The posts, copings and bar tried in the mouth and checked for accuracy of fit and retention.

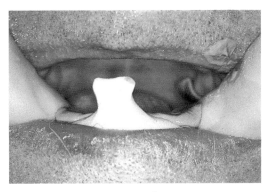

Fig 4.22 An accurate overall impression was taken.

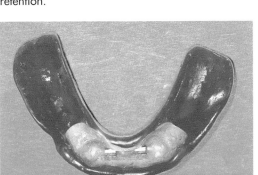

Fig 4.23 An occlusal rim constructed with Ackermann clips retained in acrylic.

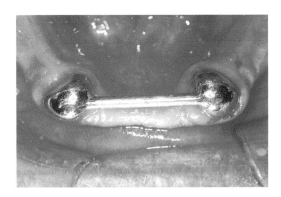

Fig 4.24 The metalwork returned to the mouth prior to taking the wax record.

tried in the mouth for accuracy of fit (Fig 4.21).

The undercut beneath the bar was blocked out with carding wax to prevent the impression material from tearing and an overall impression was taken (Fig 4.22). On removing the impression from the mouth the metalwork may be dislodged but it should accurately localize back before casting the master model.

The clips and spacers were placed on the bar, incorporated into an acrylic section that would eventually retain the overdenture, and a wax rim was constructed over this (Fig 4.23).

Having replaced the metalwork into the roots (Fig 4.24), the mandibular and maxillary wax rims were used to record the vertical dimension, incisal length, lip support and centric relation (Fig 4.25). The try-in was carried out as usual and the dentures were returned to the laboratory for processing (Fig 4.26).

At the fit stage the metalwork was

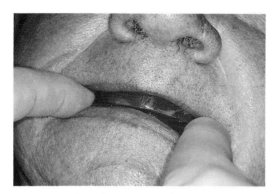

Fig 4.25 Taking the wax record.

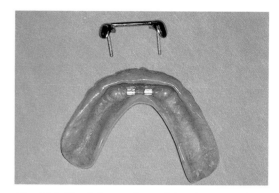

Fig 4.26 The fitting surface of the denture with Ackermann clips processed in the acrylic.

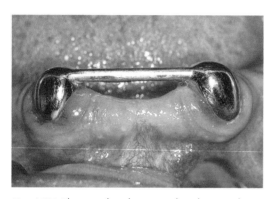

Fig 4.27 The metalwork returned to the mouth before the finished denture was tried in.

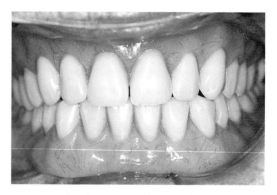

Fig 4.28 The dentures tried in. At this stage it is important to check that the mandibular denture clicks audibly into position over the Ackermann bar.

again placed in the mouth and all necessary adjustments made to the over-dentures (Figs 4.27 and 4.28). The metal-work was cleaned, dried and cemented into the roots. A light pressure should be exerted against it to prevent bounce back (Figs 4.29 to 4.31). The completed case is shown in Fig 4.32.

Another popular bar is the **Dolder bar**, also available in two types: pear-shaped, which allows a degree of resilience of movement between it and the sleeve, and the parallel bar, which allows no move-ment. Unlike the Ackermann bar, a Dolder bar cannot be bent to shape.

Tallgren (1972)[4] has confirmed practi-tioners' and patients' observations that the mandible undergoes greater resorption than the maxilla. This explains the gradual lack of retention, soreness and decreasing function which patients with full mandib-ular dentures so frequently complain of.

If conditions are favorable this prob-lem can be solved by the provision of

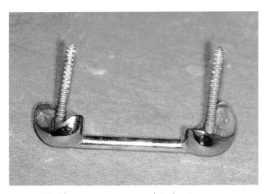

Fig 4.29 The castings were dried prior to cementation.

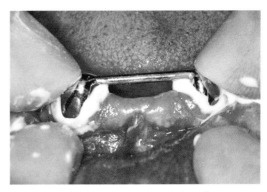

Fig 4.30 The metalwork cemented in place. It is necessary to maintain downward pressure until the cement has set: this will avoid bounce-back due to pressures set up in the root canals by the cement.

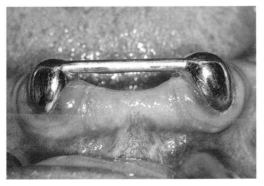

Fig 4.31 The cement was thoroughly cleaned off the metalwork and tissues.

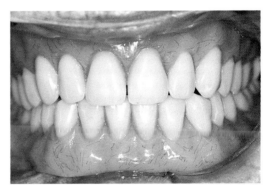

Fig 4.32 The completed work gave much improved retention and stability to the mandibular denture.

an overdenture which clips onto two implants but this is a relatively expensive and complicated procedure. It is advisable to consider keeping some mandibular teeth to retain an overdenture.

Patients often request the extraction of the last of their seemingly dispensable six mandibular anterior teeth in the mistaken belief that a full mandibular denture is the best solution to their problem.

However, careful examination and radiographs will often reveal that the two mandibular canines have relatively good bony support and could be used to retain an overdenture, which would be much more stable than a full denture. This is particularly desirable for elderly patients whose poor neuromuscular control will cause difficulty in adapting to a full mandibular denture.

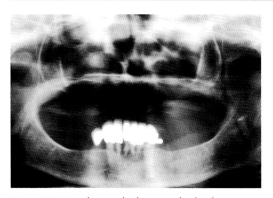

Fig 4.33 A radiograph showing the broken-down fixed partial denture of a 78-year-old female patient. Although the canines had good bone support, the incisors had very little.

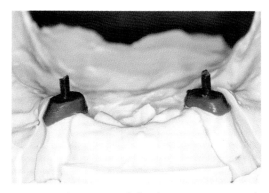

Fig 4.34 The posts and diaphragms were waxed with the diaphragms modelled flat and at right angles to the proposed path of insertion of the prosthesis.

Case 3

Figure 4.33 shows the above technique. A 78-year-old woman was complaining of loose mandibular incisors. It was decided to save the mandibular canines, which had relatively good bony support despite having suffered vertical bone loss of approximately 4 mm.

An immediate full mandibular over-denture was made, fitting over the region of the extracted incisors and decoronated canines. The root canals were filled and prepared for posts and diaphragms.

The impression was cast and the diaphragms waxed onto the posts (Fig 4.34). The extensions of the posts help in the withdrawal of the wax pattern. The surface of the wax diaphragm had been modelled flat and at right angles to the proposed path of insertion of the prosthesis and after casting these surfaces were milled to great accuracy.

It had been decided to use the **Schubiger-SB 33.01** attachment as this allows contingency planning should one of the roots be lost at a later stage. The

Schubiger-SB 33.01 precision attachment is a screwblock, constructed on the same base as a Gerber-RZ 32.02. This provides flexibility as it can be modified to accept the Gerber-RZ 32.025, the large SB 33.02 and the Dalbo-B 52089. All of these root-faced attachments allow for some contingency planning in the event of one of the roots being lost at some time in the future.

The Schubiger comes in three parts: a base with threaded screw, a hollow sleeve with shoulder, and a cap screw with shoulder. The cap screw retains the hollow sleeve when screwed onto the retention core screw.

The threaded screw bases of the Schubigers were soldered onto the gold diaphragms, ensuring that they complied with the path of insertion (Figs 4.35 to 4.37). The hollow sleeves were then screwed onto the block (Fig 4.38).

A bar system, the Dolder bar in this case (Fig 4.39), was chosen to extend between the two hollow sleeves. The bar was waxed onto the hollow

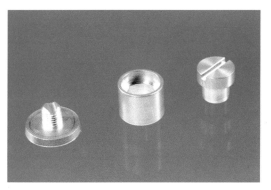

Fig 4.35 The Schubiger-SB 33.01 attachment. The three separate component parts are the base with threaded screw, a hollow sleeve with shoulder, and a cap screw with shoulder.

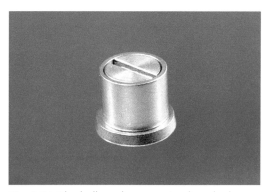

Fig 4.36 The hollow sleeve retained on the base by the cap screw secured on a threaded extension from the base.

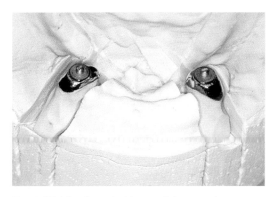

Fig 4.37 The threaded base of the attachment soldered to the diaphragms.

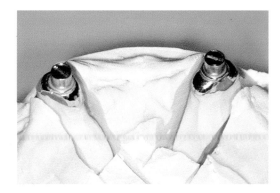

Fig 4.38 The attachments fully assembled and ready for the placing of the Dolder bar.

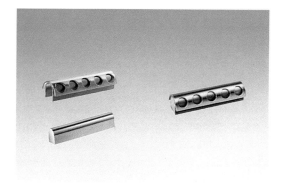

Fig 4.39 The Dolder bar attachment.

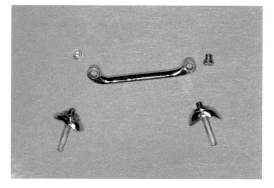

Fig 4.40 The Dolder bar soldered to the sleeves of the Schubiger attachment.

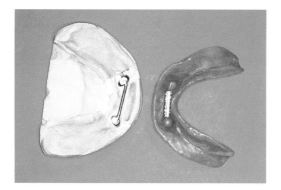

Fig 4.41 The fitting surface of the denture with the Dolder bar sleeve processed in acrylic, and the casting on the master model.

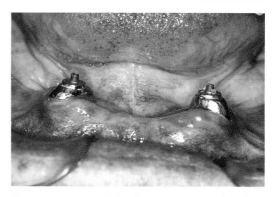

Fig 4.42 Posts and diaphragms cemented, with the threaded screw projecting from the base.

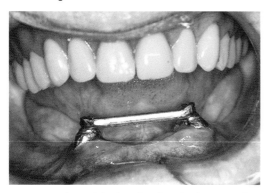

Fig 4.43 The Dolder bar fixed to the bases with the cap screw.

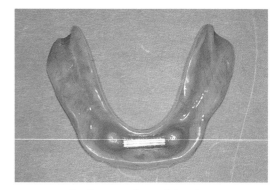

Fig 4.44 The fitting surface of the denture with the Dolder bar sleeve. The acrylic was relieved on either side of the sleeve to give flexibility.

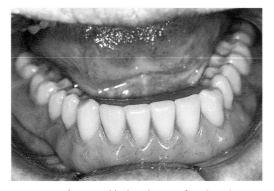

Fig 4.45 The mandibular denture fitted and giving much improved retention. Splinting the canines allowed the load to be shared, distributing forces more evenly.

sleeves and then soldered in this position. The Dolder bar matrix was then processed into the denture base (Figs 4.40 and 4.41).

Figure 4.42 shows the post and diaphragm with the threaded screw projecting, and Fig 4.43 the Dolder bar attached to the hollow sleeves and secured to the screw and base by means of the cap screw. Figure 4.44 is a view of the fitting surface of the denture with the Dolder bar sleeve localized and processed. Figure 4.45

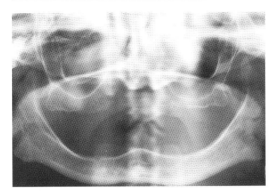

Fig 4.57 Implants were placed for this patient, as no teeth remained for the construction of an overdenture.

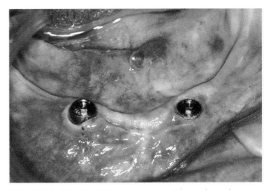

Fig 4.58 Two implants were positioned so that the bar constructed on them did not encroach on the tongue space.

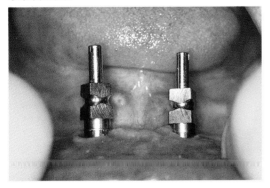

Fig 4.59 The impression copings were fully screwed down onto the fixture heads. The elongated pins will project through holes cut in the special tray constructed in the laboratory for the accurate overall impression.

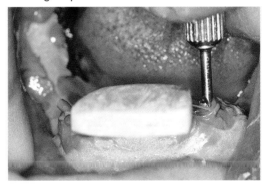

Fig 4.60 The pins were unscrewed after the impression material had set.

Case 5

An example of what is probably the simplest and most easily constructed kind of implant retained prosthesis, and the one with the most predictable results, is shown on the radiograph in Fig 4.57. An Ackermann bar and clips were used to retain an overdenture in the mandibular arch where the patient had complained of lack of retention and stability of her conventional full mandibular denture.

Two implants had been placed four months previously, and after placing healing abutments to allow tissue healing and stabilization in the immediate implant area, standard abutments were screwed onto the fixtures (Fig 4.58). These should not extend so far above the ridge as to encroach on the space available for the construction of a bar as well as a full mandibular denture of normal contour. The implants had also

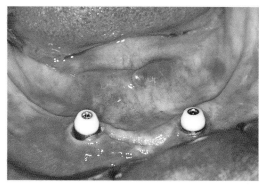

Fig 4.61 Healing caps were placed over the abutments to protect them.

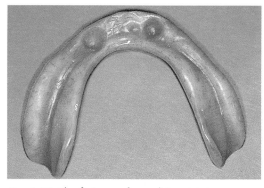

Fig 4.62 The fitting surface of the old denture was relieved to fit over the healing caps.

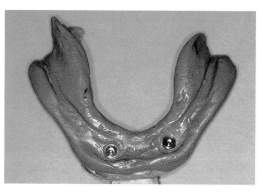

Fig 4.63 The squared copings were localized securely in the impression.

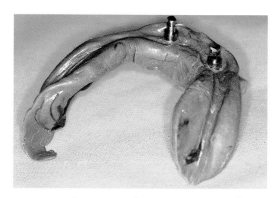

Fig 4.64 Abutment analogues were screwed into the impression copings prior to pouring the working model.

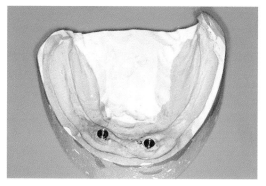

Fig 4.65 Two gold cylinders were placed on the abutment replicas.

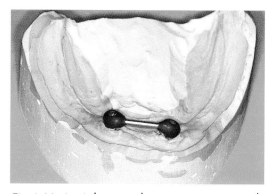

Fig 4.66 An Ackermann bar was cut to size and waxed to the abutment pins securing the gold cylinders.

been placed so as not to encroach on tongue space after construction of the bar.

Using squared impression copings and guide pins which projected through apertures in the special tray to localize the positions of the abutments, an overall impression was taken using polyether (Figs 4.59 and 4.60). Healing caps were then placed over the abutments (Fig 4.61) and the existing denture was relieved over these and relined using a soft relining material (Fig 4.62).

In the laboratory a model was produced from the impression by screwing the standard abutment analogues onto the impression copings and replacing them in the impression before pouring the model (Figs 4.63 and 4.64).

Two standard gold cylinders were placed on the abutment replicas and secured using guide pins (Fig 4.65). The Ackermann bar was cut to size and wax was applied to the abutment pins. The ends of the bar were slightly roughened and the bar was embedded in the wax pattern. The guide pins were unscrewed (Fig 4.66) and the wax pattern with the cast-on bar was invested and cast (Fig 4.67). The metalwork was finished and placed back on the model (Fig 4.68), and the fit and localization were checked carefully.

The Ackermann clips are supplied with spacers (Fig 4.69) which were placed in the top of the clip before it was placed onto the bar. The spacers remained in place during the localizing stage and after that were removed, leaving a space between the top of the clip and the top of the bar. This allows the

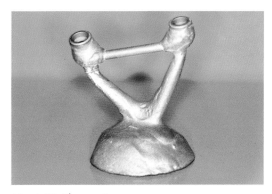

Fig 4.67 The casting.

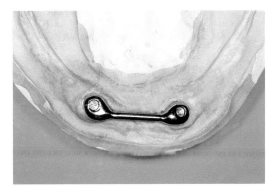

Fig 4.68 The casting finished, placed back on the model and checked for accuracy of fit.

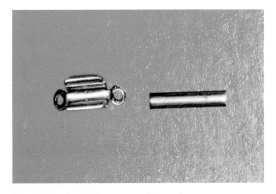

Fig 4.69 An Ackermann clip and spacer.

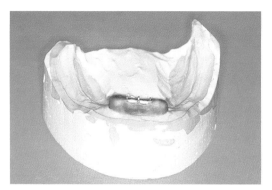

Fig 4.70 The Ackermann clips located over the bar with autopolymer acrylic resin.

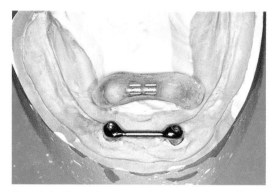

Fig 4.71 The Ackermann clips were relieved from the acrylic to allow them to spring in and out when seating or removing the denture.

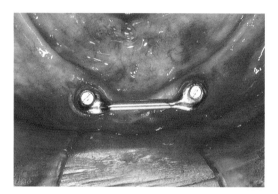

Fig 4.72 The bar was tried in the mouth and checked carefully to ensure a passive fit.

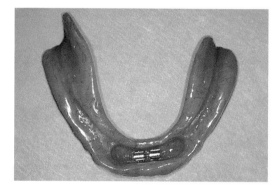

Fig 4.73 A view of the undersurface of the completed mandibular denture showing the clips and normal extension over the edentulous ridges.

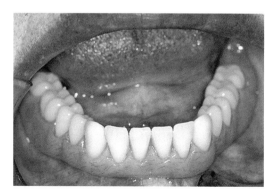

Fig 4.74 The secure mandibular denture remained seated when the mouth was opened wide, demonstrating good retention.

soft tissue to provide support while the clips and bar retain the denture. In this way the load on the implants is reduced.

The two clips and their spacers were placed on the bar. The undersurface of the bar, the sides of the clips and the gold cylinders were relieved with wax and the clips located using autopolymer acrylic resin (Fig 4.70). It is important to ensure that the retentive sides of the clips are relieved from the acrylic to allow them to spring in and out when seating or removing the denture (Fig 4.71).

The metal was tried in the patient's mouth and checked to ensure there was a passive fit (Fig 4.72). If there is a discrepancy, the patient will often feel pain as the gold screws are tightened. In this event the bar would have to be sectioned from one of the gold cylinders and re-located in the mouth using autopolymer resin, embedded in soldering investment, soldered and retried in the mouth.

Once the metalwork was found to fit accurately and passively, normal denture procedures were carried out. The fitting surface of the denture with the two clips in situ can be seen in Fig 4.73 and the completed work in Fig 4.74.

Patients sometimes complain of similar difficulties with a maxillary denture, again usually due to unretentive ridges which can affect not only retention but also the position of the maxillary anterior teeth. These, in most circumstances, have to be positioned more lingually, and shortened to reduce the displacing forces on the denture.

Case 6

Figure 4.75 shows a typical case where four implants have been placed for the retention of a bar. The metalwork was extended slightly mesially to allow an adequate thickness of metal around the cast-on Ackermann bar. Placing the bar slightly anteriorly reduced the bulk of acrylic palatally. Two small bars were placed distally to the posterior implants in order to increase the amount of retention (Fig 4.76). This procedure is possible only when implants are long and the bone quality is good.

As in all cases the metalwork was

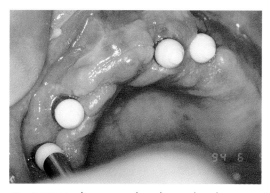

Fig 4.75 Healing caps placed over the abutments on four long implants.

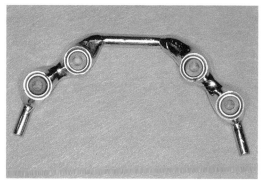

Fig 4.76 The metalwork extended forwards mesially allowing an adequate thickness of metal around the joint between the Ackermann bar and the gold cylinders. This also prevented overcontouring of the acrylic palatally.

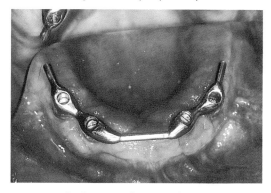

Fig 4.77 The bar must fit passively. Short extensions distally were possible because the implants were 18 and 20 mm long.

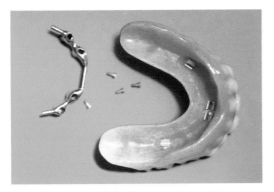

Fig 4.78 A view of the fitting surface of the denture showing four clips and the acrylic cut away in the palate.

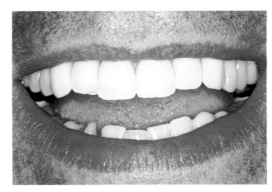

Fig 4.79 The completed overdenture offered excellent retention, allowing good positioning of the maxillary anterior teeth.

tried in and checked carefully for fit (Fig 4.77). The denture was finished and the acrylic cut back as far as possible in the palate (Fig 4.78). The completed overdenture can be seen in Fig 4.79 with the anterior teeth well positioned to maximize esthetics.

References

1 *Carr CM.* Anchored adjustable dentures. Cosmos Dent 40: 219, 1898.

2 *Bennett AG.* The vertical half-cap or bridge-work anchorage. Cosmos Dent 46: 367-369, 1904.

3 *Fossume FL.* Removable and stationary bridges. Cosmos Dent 48: 859-860, 1906.

4 *Tallgren A.* The continuing reduction of the residual alveolar ridges in complete denture wearers: A mixed longitudinal study covering 25 years. J Prosthet Dent 27: 120-132, 1972.

5 *Rangert B; Gurne J; Sullivan DY.* Mechanical aspects of a Brånemark implant connected to a natural tooth: An in vitro study. Int J Oral Maxillofac Implants 6: 177-185, 1991.

Further Reading

Barker RM; Harrison A; Ralph JP. Overdentures in General Dental Practice. London: British Dental Journal, 1993.

Brewer AA; Morrow RM. Overdentures. 2nd Edition. Saint Louis: CV Mosby, 1980.

Preiskel HW. Precision Attachments in Prosthodontics, Overdentures and Telescopic Prostheses. Vol 2. Chicago: Quintessence Publishing Co, 1985.

Preiskel HW. Overdentures Made Easy. London: Quintessence Publishing Co, 1996.

5 Auxiliary Attachments

A wide variety of attachments fall into this category, though only a few of the most significant can be described here. These are:

· Screw and tube
· Key and Keyway
· Presso-Matic or Ipsoclip
· Sectional dentures.

Screw and Tube

Screw and tube attachments consist of either two or three parts:

· A screw with a tapered head and threaded tube.
· A screw with a tapered head, collar and threaded tube (Fig 5.1).

This is one of the most versatile attachments. The assembled parts can be seen in Fig 5.2.

Cendres & Metaux (CM) attachments come in a wide range of sizes, the total length of the screw and tube varying from 5 to 8.1 mm and the diameter from 1.6 to 2 mm. The heads of the screws are elongated but, if necessary, can be shortened by 2.7 mm.

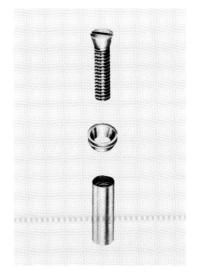

Fig 5.1
The screw and tube attachment.

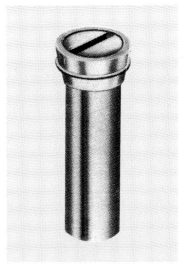

Fig 5.2 The assembled screw and tube.

Although Metaux Precieux have only a small range of sizes, these are adequate. The total length of screw and tube varies from 3.3 to 6.5 mm and the diameter from 1.7 to 2 mm. It is always advisable to use the longest screw and tube possible.

The tubes can be cast into, or soldered to, the substructure, or incorporated into extensions off a conventional retainer. The collar is cast into the superstructure and the screw with its tapered head unites the two parts.

Screw and tube attachments are useful in the following situations:

· Overcoming alignment problems
· Connecting one restoration or fixed partial denture to another
· Providing contingency planning where teeth have an unpredictable long-term prognosis
· Allowing the removal of long-span fixed partial dentures for repair and a more detailed examination of abutments or implants.

Overcoming Alignment Problems

Moderate alignment problems can sometimes be solved by the use of an interlock, Key and Keyway or telescopic crown. However, if the degree of convergence of the abutment teeth is greater, none of these is acceptable. Their use would result in an overcontouring in the cervical area because it would not be possible to house them within the normal contour of the crown.

The telescopic crown technique can also be problematic. Here the inner substructure is waxed up on the tilted abutment tooth and realigned to the same path of insertion as the other abutment or abutments, but this invariably leads to an unretentive union between substructure and superstructure.

The best solution to major alignment problems is the screw and tube.

Clinical and Laboratory Procedures

When using the screw and tube the following stages are necessary:

Stage 1

Study models are mounted on a semi-adjustable articulator using a face-bow to mount the maxillary model.

Stage 2

The abutment teeth are prepared conventionally, no attempt being made to realign the teeth to a common path of insertion. An accurate elastomeric impression is taken and centric occlusion recorded in wax. Individual temporary crowns are used at this stage.

The impression is poured in die stone and the dies sawn out and trimmed accurately. Using the centric record, the model is secured to the opposing model and mounted on an articulator. An acrylic temporary restoration is then constructed in two parts (Fig 5.3).

Stage 3

The temporary crowns are removed and the final impression is taken. The two sections of the temporary restoration are cemented onto the abutment teeth and localized together using an auto-polymer acrylic resin. Finally, the occlusion is checked carefully in both centric and eccentric movements (Fig 5.4).

Using die stone, a working model is poured from the impression, and also a further set of individual dies. This second set of dies is trimmed accurately and used to make acrylic copings which are used to record centric occlusion accurately.

Stage 4

The temporary restoration is sectioned in the mouth and the two parts removed. The acrylic copings are placed on the abutment teeth and checked to ensure that they are fully seated and out of occlusion with the opposing arch. An autopolymer resin is mixed and, when starting to gel, is placed on the occlusal surfaces of the copings. The patient then closes into centric occlusion, guided by the natural teeth (Fig 5.5).

When the resin has set the copings are removed. The two parts of the acrylic temporary restoration are placed on the prepared abutment teeth and localized together, as in Stage 3.

Having replaced the copings on the master model, this is then secured to the opposing model and plastered to the lower arm of the articulator (Fig 5.6).

Stage 5

A complete wax-up is made of the permanent fixed partial denture (Fig 5.7). The wax is heated in the distal area of the pontic and the complete screw and tube is inserted and angled slightly mesially. Keeping the head of the screw slightly

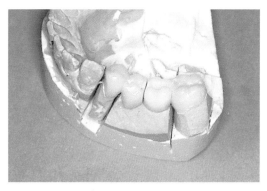

Fig 5.3 An acrylic temporary restoration was made in two parts to overcome alignment problems between molar and premolar.

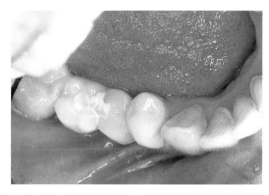

Fig 5.4 The two parts of the temporary restoration were localized in the mouth with autopolymer acrylic resin.

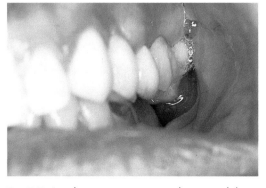

Fig 5.5 Acrylic copings were used to record the occlusion.

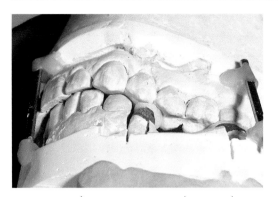

Fig 5.6 Acrylic copings were used to articulate the models.

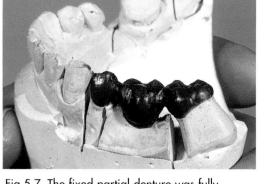

Fig 5.7 The fixed partial denture was fully waxed up.

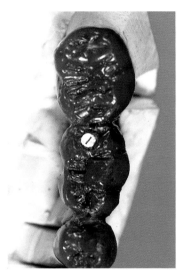

Fig 5.8 A screw and tube of suitable size was inserted into the wax pattern, angled slightly mesially.

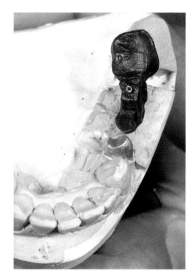

Fig 5.9 The wax pattern was cut back and angled to the same path of insertion as the mesial abutment.

out of occlusion (Fig 5.8), the wax is then cut back to produce a block in which the screw, tube and collar are left in situ. The collar (or the tapered head of the screw if a collar is not used) is completely exposed. The block is carved and angled to the same path of insertion as the mesial abutment preparation.

It is important that the location of substructure to superstructure is positive: if movement takes place between the two parts of the pontic there is a chance that the screw will work loose. To increase retention between the two parts a piece of stainless steel wire can be inserted into the wax pattern at the same angle as the mesial abutment preparation and cast onto. After casting, the wire is easily removed (Figs 5.9 and 5.10). Screw and collar are then removed prior to casting.

Using the Cendres & Metaux system it is possible to cast onto the tube. If this is the chosen technique, a fixing pin is screwed into the tube prior to investing. The fixing pin works well with yellow gold alloys, which have a low melting point, but problems can be encountered when casting onto high melting point alloys. Due to the high temperatures involved, the fixing pin oxidizes so that it can not be removed from the tube, or can be removed only with difficulty.

Where a decision has been made to solder, as in this case, the tube is removed from the wax pattern and a hole slightly smaller than the diameter of the tube is made through the wax at the base of the tube and carried through to the under-surface of the pontic. This allows the investment material to pass through more readily and simplifies the soldering technique.

When cast, the tube is placed back in the casting and soldered from the under-surface of the pontic: soldering from the occlusal surface is risky as solder may enter the threads of the tube.

The metalwork can now be finished and grooves milled in the buccal and lingual surfaces of the block to increase the retention between substructure and superstructure (Fig 5.11).

The tube is placed in the casting and soldered from the undersurface of the pontic (Fig 5.12). A plastic pin is inserted into the hole left by the removal of the stainless steel wire (Fig 5.13). The screw and collar are screwed fully into the tube and the wax-up is completed on the mesial abutment and the superstructure of the pontic (Fig 5.14).

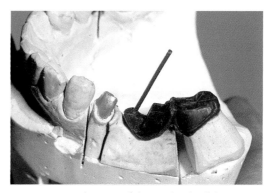

Fig 5.10 A side view of the cut back of the wax pattern and the stainless steel wire which was inserted at the same angle as the mesial abutment preparation.

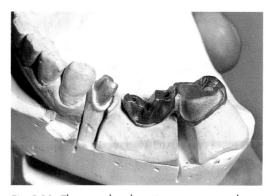

Fig 5.11 The completed casting was returned to the working model and grooves were milled in the buccal and lingual surfaces of the block.

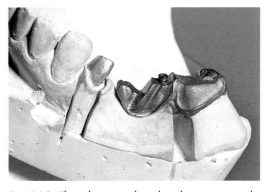

Fig 5.12 The tube was placed in the casting and soldered from the undersurface of the pontic.

69

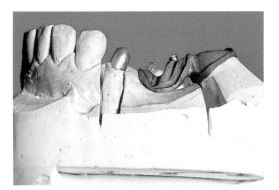

Fig 5.13 A plastic pin was inserted into the hole left by the removal of the stainless steel wire.

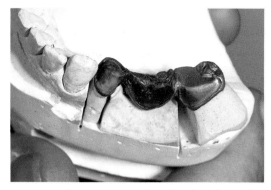

Fig 5.14 The screw was placed in the tube and the wax-up of the mesial abutment and superstructure of the pontic was completed.

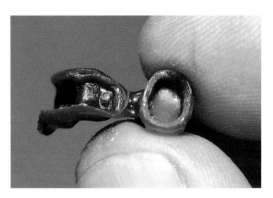

Fig 5.15 The screw was removed and the wax pattern was made ready for casting.

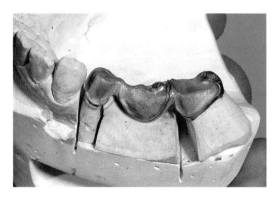

Fig 5.16 The second casting was placed on the working model and checked for accuracy of fit and localization of the screw in the tube.

The screw is then removed and the wax pattern invested (Fig 5.15), cast and finished in the usual way (Fig 5.16).

The metalwork can be tried in to check the fit and localization if desired.

Stage 6

The porcelain is applied to the metalwork and the fixed partial denture completed for insertion into the mouth (Fig 5.17).

Having tried in the fixed partial denture and again checked the margins and the occlusion, the fixed partial denture

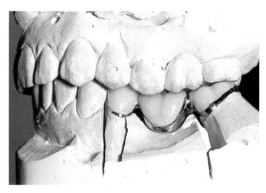

Fig 5.17 The completed fixed partial denture solved the problem of the marked misalignment of abutments.

and the abutment teeth are made ready for cementation.

The distal retainer carrying the pontic substructure is cemented first, followed by the mesial retainer and pontic super-structure. The screw with its tapered head secures the two parts.

Connecting One Restoration or Partial Denture to Another

It may be necessary to connect one fixed partial denture or retainer to another so that the stress on a connector can be reduced, or so that better support and retention are provided.

Case 1

Figure 5.18 is a labial view of a case where the patient wore a maxillary partial denture replacing 3, 6, 8, 9, 10, 12 and 13. The teeth on the denture, as well as the crowns at 7 and 11, were considerably lighter in tone than her own natural teeth. As is often the case, her desire was to have the lightest shade of tooth possible in the maxillary arch.

Figure 5.19 is a palatal view (a mirror image) and Fig 5.20 a labial view with the partial denture removed. It shows that 7 was considerably proclined in relation to the more vertical path of withdrawal of 5 and 11. The lateral incisor was also a vital tooth and the mandibular incisors had a tendency to fan out.

Because of her age the patient would not consider orthodontic treatment in order that 7 could be brought into more favorable alignment with 5 and 11. Any anterior fixed partial denture would have

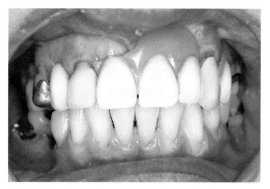

Fig 5.18 The patient presented wanting fixed partial dentures.

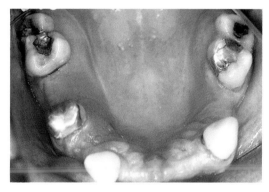

Fig 5.19 An occlusal view showing that 7 was proclined to such an extent that a common path of withdrawal with other teeth in the arch was impossible.

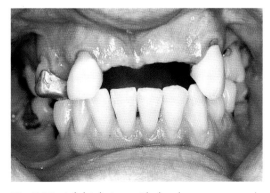

Fig 5.20 A labial view with the denture removed showing the extent of proclination.

71

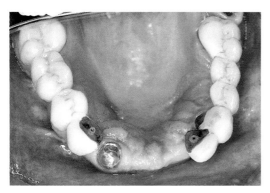

Fig 5.21 Cantilevered pontics from fixed partial dentures posteriorly allowed screw and tubes to be placed in the canine and lateral incisor positions. A gold thimble was constructed for 7.

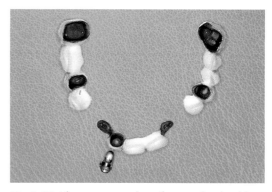

Fig 5.22 The crown made to fit over the thimble also carried the two central incisor pontics and the metal wing extensions that held the collars for the screw and tube attachment.

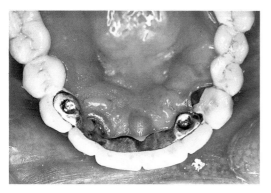

Fig 5.23 An occlusal view of the fitted anterior fixed partial denture.

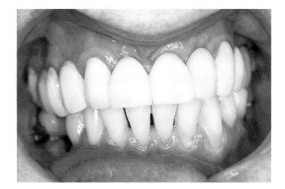

Fig 5.24 The completed case.

to rely not only on 7 for support and retention, but also on 5 and 11. These teeth were also to provide support and retention for fixed posterior partial dentures.

Some means had to be found to connect the anterior fixed partial denture with the posterior fixed partial denture. The pontics at 6 and 10 were directly cantilevered and housed the tubes for the screw and tube attachment. Pinholes for additional stability and localization were also incorporated (Fig 5.21, mirror

image). An inner gold thimble was constructed for 7 which completely covered the crown preparation underneath. This was only 0.5 mm thick, thus using the minimum amount of space.

Figure 5.22 shows the component parts of the maxillary reconstruction. It can be seen that the crown made to fit over the inner gold thimble also carries the two central incisor pontics and the metal wing extensions that house the collars for the screw and tube attachment.

72

The path of insertion for this superstructure was dictated by the preparation on 7. The pins on the wings and the pinholes in the two pontics at 6 and 10 had the same path of withdrawal.

The non-fitting surface of the inner gold thimble was highly polished and a slightly thinner cement mix was used to fix the superstructure. The two screws were then used to secure the anterior and posterior restorations.

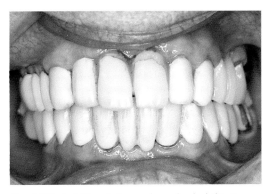

Fig 5.25 A failing full-mouth oral rehabilitation.

The placement of the inner thimble at 7 was to protect the underlying preparation in the event of the cement seal breaking down during function. Because the non-fitting surface was highly polished, the seal would fracture between the thimble and the overlying crown, enabling recementation following removal of the screws. Without the inner thimble a fracture of the cement seal might not be noticed by the patient, and this could result in rapid carious breakdown of the underlying preparation.

Figures 5.23 and 5.24 show the completed restoration, which has remained trouble free for over eighteen years.

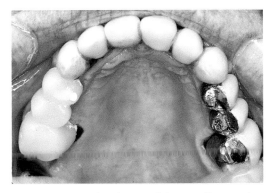

Fig 5.26 An occlusal view of the maxillary teeth.

Providing Contingency Planning

The long-term prognosis of a tooth, especially if it has a deep restoration, has been root filled or has had an apisectomy, can not be predicted. It may in some circumstances be prudent to extract a tooth where there is every likelihood of difficulties arising at some future date.

Case 2

Figures 5.25 to 5.29 show a failed

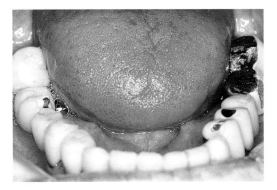

Fig 5.27 An occlusal view of the mandibular teeth.

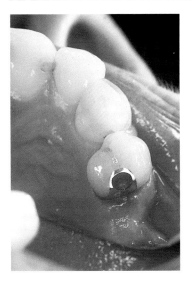

Fig 5.36
A milled
tapered
keyway in
the distal of
12.

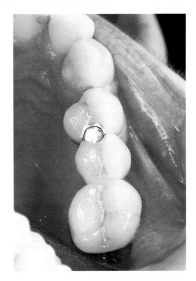

Fig 5.37
The mesial
surface of
the pontic
13 carried
a key
allowing
12 to
support the
fixed partial
denture but
not retain it.

would have to be provided while the repair was being made.

Key and Keyway

This is a passive attachment that can be constructed in the laboratory; or pre-formed plastic patterns can be used and incorporated in a wax pattern.

It is used to overcome a slight lack of parallelism of prepared abutment teeth. It is also used as a means of reducing the forces on a retainer which may have its retention compromised because the crown is short, or because it has a non-retentive core or post.

Where a fixed partial denture requires anterior support but not retention, the restoration placed in the anterior tooth does not require as much retention as that given by a full crown. Provided the restoration is large enough to house the Keyway and has sufficient retention to withstand the small forces on it, the Keyway will function well in providing the necessary anterior support.

These minor retainers, as they are called, can be intruded independently of the remainder of the fixed partial denture. If load is placed on the pontic and major retainer, the minor retainer and the abutment tooth that houses it will help to support this load.

Case 4

In Fig 5.36 a small box was prepared in the distal of the crown on 12. This tooth also had a pinned core. Having waxed up the pattern, a bur shank shaped to produce a tapered dovetail was incorporated into the wax pattern in the same long axis as the distal retainer. This was then removed and the pattern cast and finished.

The distal retainer and pontic, carrying a Key which had been waxed into the Keyway in the distal of 12, was cast and finished (Fig 5.37).

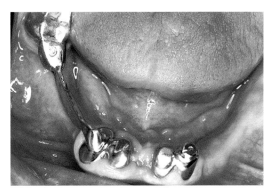

Fig 5.38 A milled bar extended from splinted gold diaphragms in 26 and 27 to a gold crown on 31, to which it was connected by a screw and tube. The bar had a small depression on the lingual surface to allow the plunger of an Ipsoclip or Presso-Matic attachment to engage it.

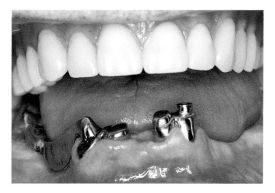

Fig 5.39 Splinted diaphragms on 23 and 24 carried an Eccentric Rothermann clip on 23.

Presso-Matic or Ipsoclip

This attachment is extremely small, enabling it to be used in confined spaces to improve the retention of dentures or even crowns. The author prefers to increase the retention of crowns by other means, but this attachment can be very useful for overdentures. It has been likened in its action to a door catch: a plunger housed in one section is activated by a spring which engages a corresponding depression in the other section.

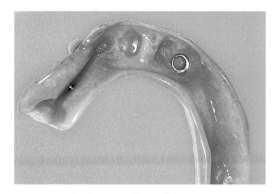

Fig 5.40 The fitting surface of the overdenture showing the plunger of the attachment lingually in the first molar region.

Case 5

Figures 5.38 and 5.39 show a bar extending from 31 to 27. The depression is located in the lingual aspect of the bar and the attachment within the lingual flange of the mandibular denture (Fig 5.40). The retention was supplemented by the Eccentric Rothermann attachment on 23. The completed work is shown in Fig 5.41.

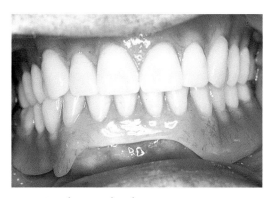

Fig 5.41 The completed case.

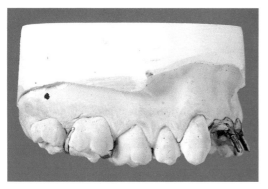

Fig 5.42 Wiptam split wire posts were angled slightly anteriorly to the mesial cervical undercuts of 6 and 10. Clasps on 2 and 15 passively engaged the distal undercuts only.

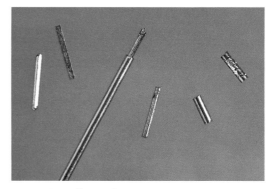

Fig 5.43 Half-round Wiptam wire was spot-welded together to form a post of 1.5 mm in diameter, onto which the chrome-cobalt base was cast.

Sectional Dentures

The majority of edentulous spaces are restored with a chrome-cobalt or all-acrylic denture. Compared with fixed partial dentures, the standard partial denture is far cheaper, does not involve major tooth preparation and restores the missing soft tissue. It does however have its disadvantages:

- Retention can be a problem, particularly in the Kennedy Class IV situation.
- The anterior flange tends to drop, making it feel very insecure.
- Conventional clasps are esthetically unacceptable, particularly gingivally approaching clasps.

The sectional denture is made in two parts: a chrome-cobalt base and a removable acrylic flange with teeth. This type of denture overcomes problems of retention and esthetics.

The construction of the sectional denture is similar to that of the conventional chrome-cobalt partial denture. The main differences are the clasps, the method of retaining the acrylic flange, and the flange itself.

Case 6

In Fig 5.42 the chrome-cobalt base had been cast. Incorporated into the casting were Wiptam split posts, angled slightly anteriorly to the mesial cervical undercuts on 6 and 10.

These posts were made by placing two pieces of Wiptam half-round wire (0.75 by 1.5 mm) in a stainless steel tube having an internal diameter of 1.5 mm (Fig 5.43). One end was left to protrude beyond the end of the tube and was then spot welded. The two were aligned into the wax pattern and cast onto.

The clasps engaged the distal undercuts of the abutment teeth. The chrome-cobalt base was seated with a distal path of insertion, the clasps at this stage having

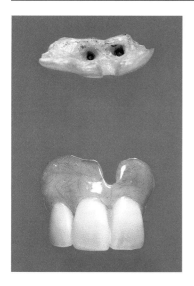

Fig 5.44 Stainless steel tubes with an internal diameter of 1.5 mm were processed in the acrylic flange, engaging the split posts and holding the two parts together.

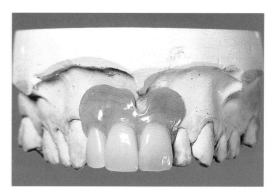

Fig 5.45 The acrylic flange engaged the mesial undercuts on 6 and 10.

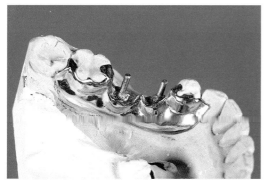

Fig 5.46 No clasps were used in this case: there were natural undercuts lingually on 18 and 21. The Wiptam split posts were angled buccally.

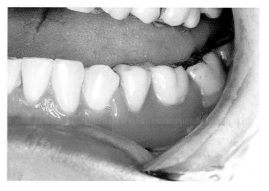

Fig 5.47 The acrylic flange engaged in the approximal cervical undercuts of 18 and 21.

passive retention only. Two stainless steel tubes engaged the split posts and were processed into the acrylic flange. This provided good retention between the acrylic flange and the chrome-cobalt base (Fig 5.44).

The acrylic flange was extended to engage the mesiocervical undercuts on 6 and 10 (Fig 5.45) and it had an anterior path of insertion guided by the split posts. The denture was retained securely in the mouth by using opposing undercuts, that is the distobuccal surfaces of 2 and 15 and also the mesiocervical surfaces of 6 and 10.

Over a period of time wear will take place between the split posts and the tubes, resulting in a loss of retention between the flange and the chrome-cobalt base. Retention can be reactivated by using a scalpel to prise the two split posts slightly apart.

Case 7

In Fig 5.46 the same principle of using opposing undercuts had been followed. There was no blocking out of the undercuts on the lingual surfaces of the model during construction of the chrome-cobalt base. The plate was seated with a lingual path of insertion.

The two Wiptam split posts were angled slightly bucally in relation to the approximal buccocervical undercuts at 18 and 21. The acrylic flange, therefore, was seated with a buccal path of insertion, guided and retained by the two Wiptam split posts, and engaged the approximal buccocervical undercuts of 18 and 21 (Fig 5.47).

6 Milling Using a Precision Parallelometer

The milling of crowns is a precise procedure for creating bracing, ledges and rests in full or partial veneer crowns which serve to retain conventional removable partial dentures.

Milling bracing ledges on retainers housing certain precision attachments, in free-end saddle situations, will reduce the forces transferred to the attachments and thus protect them from leverage which would decrease their retention. The bracing arm extends from the framework of the partial denture and accurately fits the milled bracing ledges on the retainers.

The following attachments require such support:

McCollum (MP)
T-123 (MP)
Biloc (CM)
Mini-Conex (CM)
Crismani (CM)
Snap-Attachment (CM)
PT-Snap (CM)
Regulex (CM)
Conex (CM)
Ceka.

Milling is useful in the following situations:

· For rest seats and ledges in anterior and posterior crowns to give support and bracing to a removable partial denture.
· For laboratory-cast bars used to retain a removable partial denture.
· For extended platforms off fixed partial denture retainers which house screw and tube attachments (MP and CM), used when abutments have a conflicting path of withdrawal (see page 66).
· For the root faces of diaphragms to receive attachments to retain overdentures (see page 53).

Milling Process

Case 1

The patient in Fig 6.1 presented with 2, 6 to 11, and 19 to 22 standing. His main concern was his intolerance of all the conventional mandibular removable partial dentures that had been made for him over a period of many years. It was decided that the remaining heavily filled mandibular teeth could be used for the support and retention of a precision

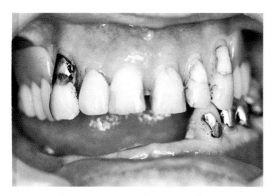

Fig 6.1 The patient's mouth prior to the commencement of treatment.

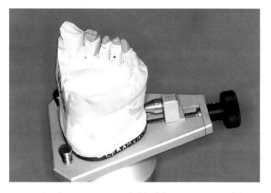

Fig 6.2 The master model held in an orientable model holder.

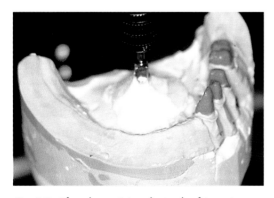

Fig 6.3 After determining the path of insertion, a transmission nut was plastered to the model.

attachment-retained denture. The milling of the crowns and provision of an extended bracing arm would be an integral part of the treatment.

The procedure for milling is as follows:

Stage 1

Secure the master model to the model holder (Fig 6.2). With an analysing rod held in the model analyser, determine the path of insertion – usually governed by the long axis of the preparations.

Stage 2

Having determined the path of insertion, drill a 6-mm hole in the floor of the model where it will not interfere with the construction of the restoration.

Stage 3

Insert a transmission nut and pin into the surveying or drilling arm. Lower the arm so that the nut seats into the previously drilled 6-mm hole. Use either plaster or autopolymer resin to secure the pin and nut to the model. When the medium has set, release the chuck holding the transmission pin and nut and raise the arm of the surveyor (Fig 6.3).

Stage 4

Remove the model from the holder and replace the model holder with the milling block on the parallelometer. Use petroleum jelly or another separating medium on the base of the master model and milling block. Reinsert the transmission pin into the chuck of the drilling spindle and locate the milling block directly underneath the master model (Fig 6.4).

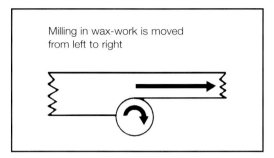

Diag 6.1

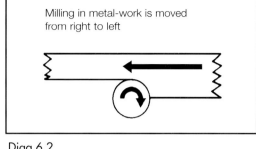

Diag 6.2

Mix some plaster, place it on the milling block and lower the master model into the plaster (Fig 6.5). This technique allows the parallelometer to be used for two or more cases at a time.

Stage 5

Remove the split cast and place the master model back on the articulator. Wax up the wax patterns. It is desirable to do the basic milling on the wax patterns, particularly when working on thick sections. This will ultimately save time and materials. Very thin sections, however, are best milled in metal as the breaking strength of the wax may be too low.

Stage 6

Remove the master model with the wax patterns from the articulator and place the model into the split cast base back on the parallelometer.

There are two methods of rough milling or carving the wax patterns. The first is to use Komet Square Wax Cutters (354.10 ISO, ref nos 018 and 012). Place the cutter in the handpiece and begin milling, using a slow speed with little pressure. The direction of the milling must be the same as the object to be milled, that is left to right (Diag 6.1). This will leave the surface of the wax smooth, with no wax chips left to adhere to the wax pattern.

The second method of producing a rough milling or carving is to use the Variotherm wax-up unit (Fig 6.6). The correct temperature (which depends on room temperature and the melting point of the wax) must first be set: it should be just hot enough to melt the wax. The Variotherm is then moved around the areas to be milled. The melted wax must continually be wiped off the heated rod.

When the rough milling is completed, invest and cast the wax pattern or patterns.

Stage 7

Divest and clean the castings, and check and finish the margins. Replace the master model, with castings in place, on the parallelometer; insert a bur into the chuck and lower it to make contact with the occlusal surface of the castings.

The bur must be sticky waxed to the casting (Fig 6.7) and the main connector block of the parallelometer raised until the casting is clear of the die on the

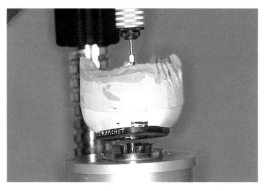 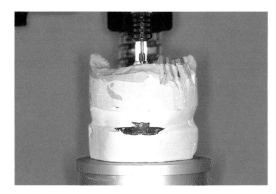

Fig 6.4-6.5 Using the transmission nut and pin, the model was lowered into plaster which had been placed on the milling block.

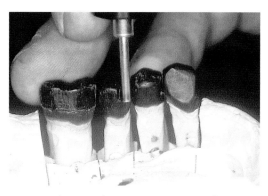

Fig 6.6 The Variotherm wax-up unit used to produce the basic milling.

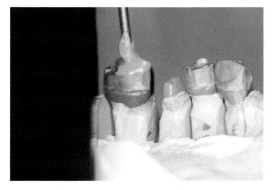

Fig 6.7 The castings were placed on the master model on the parallelometer and a bur held in the parallelometer was sticky waxed to each casting.

master model. Remove the master model from the parallelometer.

A duplicate die can be inserted into the casting, or the fitting surface lightly coated with petroleum jelly. Mix a small amount of plaster and place on the coated surface of the milling block. Lower the casting into the soft plaster, keeping the areas to be milled clear of it. This technique prevents any damage to the master model (Fig 6.8).

Stage 8

Start milling by using the largest steel cutter (Gaerny 025) and guide the milling block freehand. The optimum efficiency of the cutters is achieved between 3,000 and 5,000 rpm, working with as little pressure as possible, using Cajuputi oil for lubrication and cooling. The metalwork is moved from right to left (Fig 6.9), the opposite of what is done when milling wax patterns (Diag 6.2).

When the milling of the walls of the crown is complete, mill the grooves

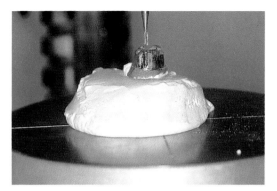

Fig 6.8 The individual castings were lowered into the plaster on the milling block.

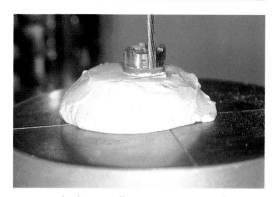

Fig 6.9 The basic milling was commenced.

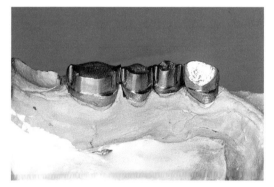

Fig 6.10 The milled surfaces were polished, and grooves were cut interproximally.

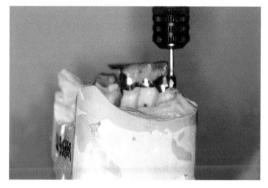

Fig 6.11 The patrix of a PR attachment was localized on the parallelometer to the mesial surface of 22.

in the distal and mesial surfaces. To determine the diameter of the grooves, measure the thickness of the walls of the crown. If, for example, the wall thickness is 0.8 mm, allowing a minimum wall thickness of 0.2 mm at the groove leaves 0.6 mm for milling the groove. The depth of the groove should be equal to half the drill diameter: therefore select a cutter of 1.2 mm maximum diameter.

Maillefer round-end Steiger cutters are used for milling the grooves.

Stage 9

Polish the milled surfaces with emery polishing paper (no 2|0 424) held in a mandrel (Fig 6.10).

In Case 1, the crowns on the mandibular left canine and premolars were splinted together with sticky wax. A PR attachment (MP) was chosen to retain the removable partial denture. Its patrix was held in the appropriate mandrel on the parallelometer and the attachment localized to the mesial surface of 22 (Fig 6.11).

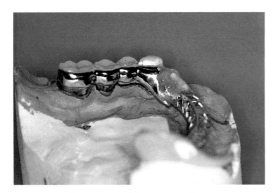

Fig 6.12 The matrix of the PR attachment was placed on the patrix and localized to the chrome-cobalt framework with autopolymer acrylic resin.

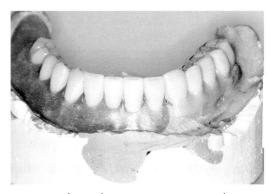

Fig 6.13 The teeth were set up on a wax base.

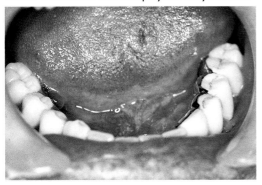

Fig 6.14 The crowns and denture were tried in.

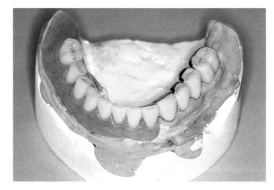

Fig 6.15 The finished crowns and denture on the master model.

The metalwork was embedded in soldering investment and the attachment soldered to the retainer; the porcelain was then applied to the metalwork. A partial chrome-cobalt framework was cast and the matrix of the PR attachment was placed on the patrix and localized to this framework with autopolymer resin (Fig 6.12).

The teeth were set up on a wax base (Fig 6.13) and tried in the mouth to check the esthetics and centric record (Fig 6.14). Finally, the denture was finished (Figs 6.15 and 6.16) and the crowns and denture fitted in the mouth (Figs 6.17 and 6.18).

At a later date the patient requested that the maxillary arch be restored, having been very happy with the results in the mandibular arch. 2 and 6 to 11 were prepared for porcelain-fused to metal crowns and PR attachments (MP) were used to retain the removable partial maxillary denture. The lateral incisor and canine on both sides were splinted.

The metalwork for the crowns and the

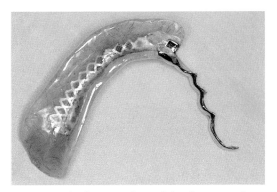

Fig 6.16 The fitting surface of the denture with the PR attachment processed in acrylic.

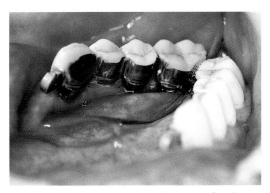

Fig 6.17-6.18 The crowns and denture fitted in the mouth.

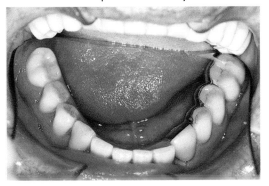

Fig 6.18

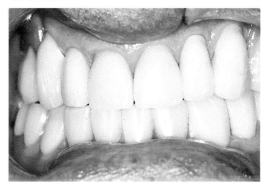

Fig 6.19 The maxillary arch was restored with splinted crowns and a denture retained by two PR attachments.

partial chrome-cobalt denture framework was cast and the attachments were localized to the distal surfaces of 6 and 11 and soldered into position. The matrix of the PR attachment was placed on the patrix and localized to the partial denture with autopolymer resin. The fit of the castings and the localization of the partial denture was verified at try-in.

The porcelain was applied to the retainers and the denture set up. This was again tried in the mouth to check the centric record and esthetics before finally processing the denture and fitting the completed work in the mouth (Fig 6.19).

Case 2

Figure 6.20 is a preoperative view of a patient who had been involved in a road traffic accident, resulting in the loss of all the maxillary incisors, as well as a considerable amount of soft tissue and bone in that area.

As the soft tissue loss was too great to allow the construction of a conventional partial denture, it was decided to place a bar and make a removable

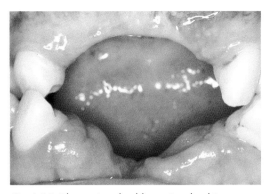

Fig 6.20 The patient had been involved in a road traffic accident, losing teeth and much soft tissue and bone.

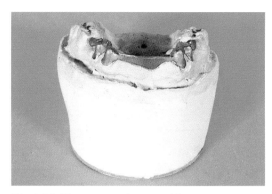

Fig 6.21 The cast retainers and bar.

prosthesis to replace the missing teeth and soft tissue. The bar was made by trimming a piece of plastic 1 mm thick to the contour of the ridge; attaching it to the wax patterns and then casting (Fig 6.21).

Figure 6.22 shows a bur shank in the chuck of a parallelometer, waxed to the flat labial surface of the cast bar. Plaster was mixed and placed on the table of the parallelometer; the casting was then lowered into the plaster. When set, the bar was milled perfectly smooth (Fig 6.23).

Porcelain was then applied to the metalwork of the retainers (Fig 6.24). On the palatal surface and at the top of the bar two tapered grooves were cut in the lateral incisor positions.

A Presso-Matic auxiliary attachment was used further to supplement the retention. The plunger and spring were removed from the attachment, the housing placed in the center of the palatal surface of the milled bar, and a sleeve waxed up around the bar incorporating

the Presso-Matic housing. The wax sleeve was then removed from the bar, the Presso-Matic housing was removed from the wax pattern, and the pattern was invested and cast.

After casting, the Presso-Matic housing was placed in the cast sleeve and soldered. The plunger and spring were replaced in the attachment. Occlusal indicator or colloidal graphite was painted on the palatal surface of the milled bar and the cast sleeve with the Presso-Matic attachment was seated on the bar.

When the sleeve was removed a tracing in the indicating medium was left by the plunger. At the top of the tracing a tapering groove was cut so that, when the sleeve was placed on the bar and seated, the plunger would be depressed more readily.

At the base of the tracing an indentation was milled with a bur so that, when the sleeve was fully seated, the plunger would engage in the milled depression (Fig 6.25).

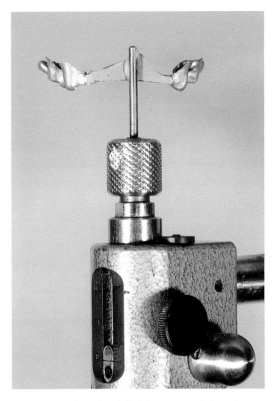

Fig 6.22 A bur shank held in a parallelometer and sticky waxed to the bar.

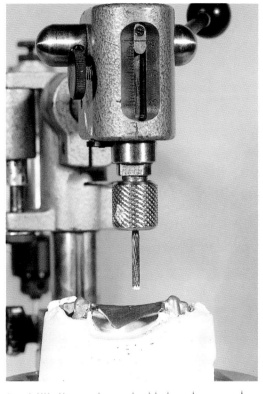

Fig 6.23 The casting embedded in plaster on the milling table, and the milled bar.

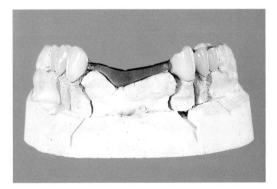

Fig 6.24 Porcelain was applied to the retainers and pontics.

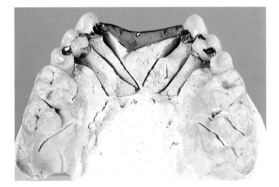

Fig 6.25 The palatal surface of the milled bar showing the milled grooves and the depression to receive the plunger of the Presso-Matic attachment.

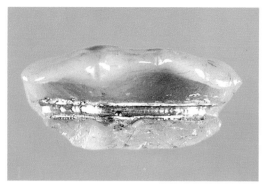

Fig 6.26 A view of the fitting surface of the denture with the cast gold sleeve processed in the acrylic. The plunger of the Presso-Matic attachment shows palatally.

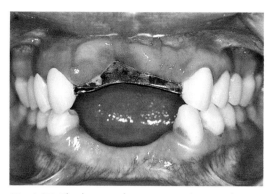

Fig 6.27 The bar ready to receive the prosthesis after cementation of the crowns.

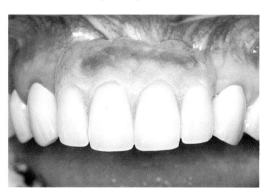

Fig 6.28 The prosthesis inserted over the bar.

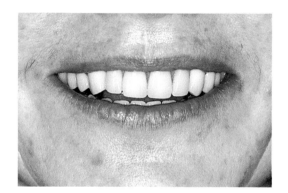

Fig 6.29 The final appearance.

The removable prosthesis was set up and waxed at the same time, incorporating the cast sleeve. This was tried in the mouth to check esthetics and localization before proceeding to the final fitting. The fitting surface of the denture with the cast sleeve processed in the acrylic and the plunger of the Presso-Matic showing palatally can be seen in Fig 6.26.

The crown and bar were first cemented in place (Fig 6.27); the denture was then inserted over the bar (Fig 6.28). Figure 6.29 shows the final appearance of the restoration.

The author would like to thank Arshad Ali, Consultant in Restorative Dentistry at Glasgow Dental Hospital and School for providing the clinical photographs used in this case.

7 The Use of Precision Attachments with Implants

There is no doubt that, thanks to the work of Brånemark and other leading implantologists, dentistry is set to take a quantum leap in the next decade. Both patients and clinicians are now becoming aware of the applications and long-term benefits of implants.

Implants are not, of course, a panacea. Not all partially or totally edentulous patients can benefit from them, though as a result of implants many can again enjoy an unimagined level of dental health and comfort. In many cases the part played by precision attachments in achieving this goal is great.

Having decided, after careful consideration, that a patient is a suitable candidate for implants, meticulous planning is essential if the result is to be successful. However, it is outside the scope of this book to describe in detail all stages in the prosthetic management of cases involving implants.

The concept of osseointegration is now well established: nevertheless it has not always been possible to provide patients with restorations that are both functional and esthetically pleasing. A successful implant depends in part on the presence of a sufficient thickness and density of bone. Where bone volume is inadequate, techniques such as ridge augmentation and sinus lifts are sometimes used but they are not routine in general dental practice, and they further complicate treatment for the patient.

In this chapter I shall attempt to show how precision attachments can be used to achieve functional esthetic restorations which otherwise would be difficult, if not impossible; and how they also provide contingency support during the removal and repair of restorations.

Treatment Planning

Implants should always be placed with the design of the final prosthesis in mind. Unfortunately, due to bone resorption patterns, they are often placed with less than ideal angulation in relation to each other and to adjacent natural teeth which might be included in the rehabilitation. Manufacturers have, to some extent, overcome this problem by producing angled abutments to compensate for the lack of parallelism in some but not all cases.

Clinicians sometimes try to solve the problem by placing additional implants, in order to gain extra support for the new prosthesis. However, it is often impossible to do this in the maxilla.

Precision attachments enable the dentist to overcome alignment and withdrawal difficulties; they are also a means whereby stress distribution is made more favorable in such circumstances. This is particularly important where implants are not vertical, or are shorter than would be ideal for the particular case in hand.

Lindquist *et al* (1988)[1] found that, along with poor plaque control, the excessive horizontal forces of occlusion on osseointegrated implants was the main cause of bone loss around fixtures. Lekholm (1983)[2] also stated that, when occlusion was poor, loads and stresses were distributed unevenly, resulting in the resorption and loosening of implants.

To avoid harmful stresses having a destructive effect on the bone around implants, the dentist has either to place more implants or, alternatively, include in the rehabilitation some or all of the natural teeth that remain in the patient's mouth (provided that these are healthy and well supported by bone). Although we do not have decades of corroborative research to support the idea that implants and teeth can in some circumstances be successfully combined, recent papers tend to support this view.[3] If we accept this evidence, the restorative options for the clinician are increased.

Where all implants and teeth are splinted and reconstruction circumvents the arch, lateral forces are greatly reduced, making it possible, in such ideal circumstances, to reduce the number of implants. It is not always necessary to use precision attachments when splinting implants, or teeth and implants. However, the author has found that, in the maxillary arch in particular, they facilitate such reconstructions and maximize esthetic results, especially when it is desirable that the reconstruction circumvents the arch.

Case Studies

There follows a description of the use of precision attachments, in conjunction with the EsthetiCone abutment and the Steri-Oss PME abutment, to overcome alignment problems between implants and teeth. It will also be shown how they can be used to facilitate the removal of a prosthesis so that the implant can be inspected, and normal maintenance and repair can be carried out more easily.

Overdentures supported by implants have been dealt with in Chapter 4. This chapter describes mainly the use of precision attachments in combination with implants for the treatment of the partially edentulous, though two of the cases were edentulous patients.

EsthetiCone Abutments

The EsthetiCone abutment (Fig 7.1) has an overall height of 6.7 mm and the abutment collars are either 1, 2 or 3 mm in height so that marginal placement can be varied to give the best esthetic results. The interocclusal space must be sufficient to accommodate the height of the abutment as well as the superstructure, otherwise it cannot be used. The Mirus

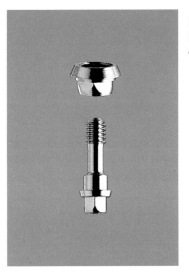

Fig 7.1 The EsthetiCone abutment.

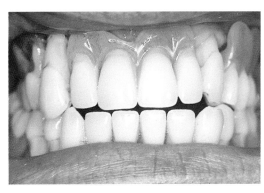

Fig 7.2 The patient's appearance when presenting for treatment.

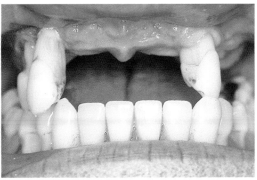

Fig 7.3 Only three maxillary teeth remained and the patient was psychologically attached to these.

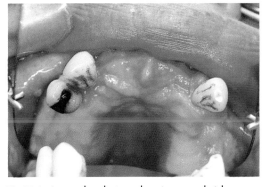

Fig 7.4 An occlusal view showing good ridge form.

Cone, a similar but shorter abutment, can be used to overcome this problem.

Case I

Figures 7.2 to 7.4 show the remaining maxillary teeth of a middle aged man who had a particular aversion to their loss. The maxillary left canine was unrestored and vital and had lost little of its bony support. The retention of this tooth would give the patient some proprioception in the maxillary arch and would also help

in positioning the maxillary implants correctly. It was, therefore, decided that it be retained and incorporated into the design of the maxillary arch rehabilitation in such a way that, were there ever to be a problem relating to the tooth, its extraction would cause minimal disruption to the reconstruction.

The maxillary right canine and first premolar were extracted and added to the existing partial maxillary denture. After a period of healing, implants were inserted

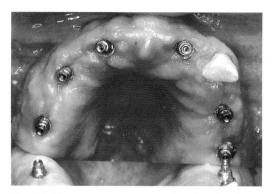

Fig 7.5 The canine was retained and EsthetiCone abutments were placed on the six implants.

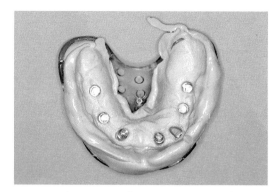

Fig 7.6 Abutment analogues were screwed onto the impression copings and carefully replaced in the impression.

at 3, 5, 7, 10, 13 and 14 and left for six months to integrate. EsthetiCone abutments were placed on these implants after healing abutments had been in position for approximately five weeks (Fig 7.5).

Transfer copings were placed on the abutments and an overall impression was taken in silicone, after the preparation of the canine for a full-bonded porcelain crown. Temporary healing caps were placed on the EsthetiCone abutments. These help to maintain the patency of the tissues until it is time to fit the final restoration.

A centric relation record was taken, as well as an accurate impression of the opposing arch. At this stage a face-bow and protrusive and lateral records were also taken to facilitate accurate mounting on a semiadjustable articulator.

In the laboratory the technician screwed abutment analogues onto the impression copings, which were then replaced in the impression. Care must be taken that these are fully seated to avoid errors (Fig 7.6). Prior to pouring up the model, an elastomeric silicone material

was syringed around the abutment analogues (Fig 7.7). This material is particularly beneficial when these are below the level of the soft tissue, which invariably leads to the soft tissue slightly overhanging the margins of the abutment analogues. This can cause problems when screwing the gold cylinders onto them. Use of the silicone overcomes this difficulty as its flexibility facilitates placement of the gold cylinders (Fig 7.8).

The models were mounted on a semiadjustable articulator using the records supplied. Temporary cylinders (Figs 7.9 and 7.10) were screwed onto the master model and reduced in height to prevent interference with the occlusion.

A wax-up of the maxillary arch was completed using acrylic stock teeth; at the same time the temporary cylinders were covered with wax (Fig 7.11). This was then duplicated and a stone model was produced (Fig 7.12). A vacuum-formed matrix was pulled down onto the duplicate model (Figs 7.13 and 7.14).

The wax was boiled off the master model, leaving the temporary cylinders

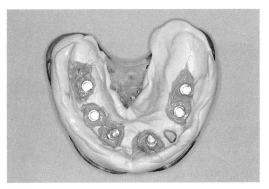

Fig 7.7 An elastomeric silicone material was syringed around the abutment analogues.

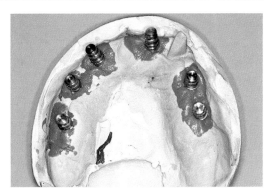

Fig 7.8 A view of the completed master model.

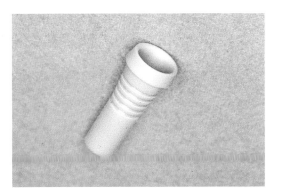

Fig 7.9-7.10 The temporary cylinders.

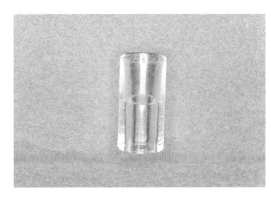

Fig 7.10

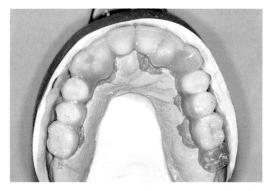

Fig 7.11 Temporary cylinders were placed on the abutment replicas and the maxillary arch was waxed up using acrylic stock teeth.

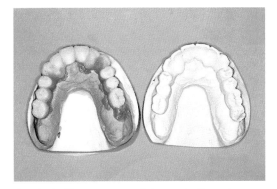

Fig 7.12 The master model was duplicated.

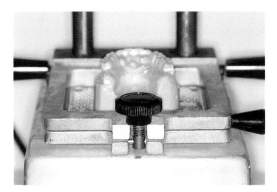

Fig 7.13 The duplicated model was placed on the vacuum former platform.

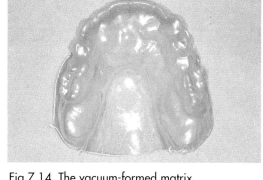

Fig 7.14 The vacuum-formed matrix.

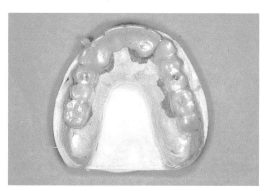

Fig 7.15 The wax was boiled off the master model leaving the temporary cylinders in place. The vacuum formed matrix was filled with autopolymer acrylic resin and placed on the master model.

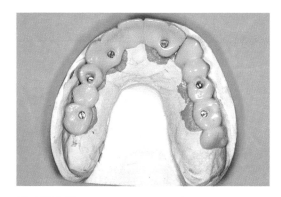

Fig 7.16 The temporary restorations were trimmed and polished.

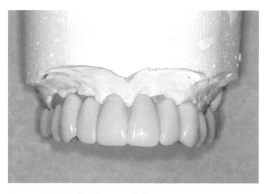

Fig 7.17 A labial view of the temporary restorations.

in place. The openings of these were filled with wax so that the dentin-colored autopolymer acrylic resin, used to make the temporary restorations, did not enter and prevent them being unscrewed.

The vacuum formed matrix was filled with autopolymer resin and placed on the master model, on which the temporary cylinders had been screwed into position (Fig 7.15). When set, the temporary restoration was trimmed and polished (Figs 7.16 and 7.17).

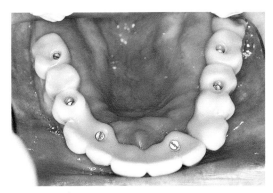

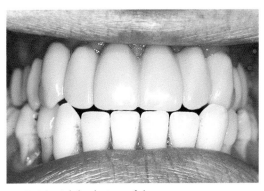

Fig 7.18 The temporary restorations were inserted in the mouth and retained by gold screws.

Fig 7.19 A labial view of the temporary restoration.

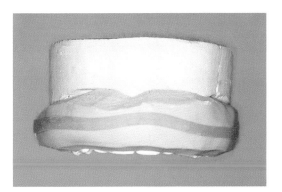

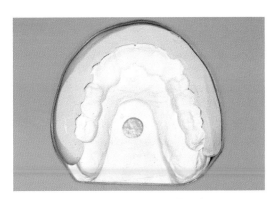

Fig 7.20-7.21 Before the temporary restorations were fitted a key of the labial and buccal surfaces was taken. During the waxing of the metalwork this was used as a guide to the correct positioning of the anterior teeth.

The temporary acrylic restorations were placed in the patient's mouth after first removing the temporary healing caps and temporary crown on the canine. They were secured in position by gold screws (Figs 7.18 and 7.19).

This type of provisional restoration offers definite advantages to the clinician. It functions as a template for the final restoration and is thus a communicative tool between patient and technician. It allows transitional loading where the quality of bone is not good. It enables the occlusion and anterior guidance to be refined, and also the phonetics.

Prior to the temporary restoration being fitted, a key of the labial and buccal surfaces of the restoration seated on the master model was taken with a silicone impression material. This key was used as a guide to the wax-up of the metalwork at the next stage (Figs 7.20 and 7.21).

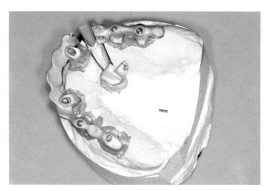

Fig 7.22 The metalwork disassembled.

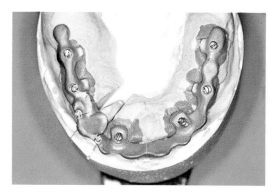

Fig 7.23 The metalwork assembled.

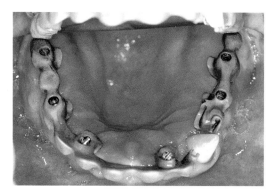

Fig 7.24 The metalwork retained by the EsthetiCone abutments was first screwed in place.

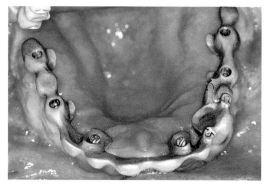

Fig 7.25 The metalwork for the crown was tried in and the fit checked carefully. Radiographs can be taken at this stage to confirm the accuracy of fit of the castings.

The design of the metalwork allowed for removal of the crown on 11, should the need arise at some future date. The metalwork extended from the EsthetiCone abutment at 3 to the one at 10 adjacent to the canine. Incorporated distally at 10 was the matrix of a Stern Tube-lock attachment. On the patient's left side the metalwork extended forwards from the abutments on that side to the 12 pontic distal to 11. This also had a Stern Tube-lock matrix mesially, and the tube of a screw and tube precision attachment in the lingual and middle of the same pontic. The metalwork for the crown incorporated the patrix of the Stern Tube-lock both mesially and distally, and the short wing and screw aperture that covered the tube in the pontic at 12 (Figs 7.22 and 7.23).

The metalwork was tried in the patient's mouth: it must fit passively and accurately (Figs 7.24 to 7.26). The temporary acrylic restorations were replaced and the ceramic work completed in the laboratory. Figures 7.27 and 7.28 show the

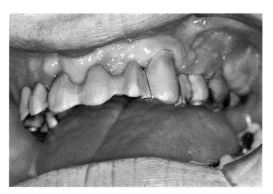

Fig 7.26 The metalwork for the canine is fully seated, linking the metalwork on either side. The screw was inserted through the extended wing on the crown into the tube incorporated in 12.

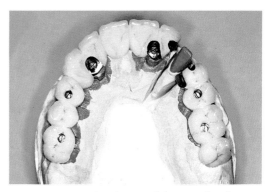

Fig 7.27 An occlusal view of the completed restorations before the placement of the crown.

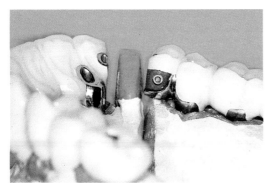

Fig 7.28 A close-up of the interlocks in the distal of 10 and mesial of 12, and the threaded tube in the lingual aspect of 12.

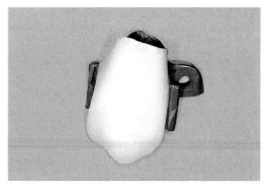

Fig 7.29 The canine crown showing the interlock patrices fitted mesially and distally, and the wing extension that would accommodate the screw.

fixed partial dentures before the placement of the crown (Figs 7.29 and 7.30).

Figures 7.31 and 7.32 show the contour of the crowns and pontics and Fig 7.33 the fitting surface.

The completed restorations were tried in and, once fit, esthetics, occlusion and phonetics were established as acceptable, were secured using the gold screws in the EsthetiCone abutments, and the crown on the canine was cemented (Figs 7.34 to 7.37).

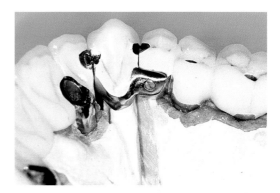

Fig 7.30 The crown fully seated on the model with the screw inserted into the threaded tube in 12.

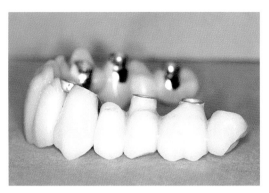

Fig 7.31 The buccal contour of the completed restoration on the left side.

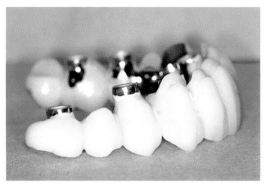

Fig 7.32 The buccal contour of the completed restoration on the right side.

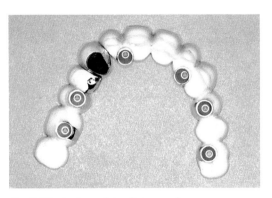

Fig 7.33 A view of the fitting surfaces.

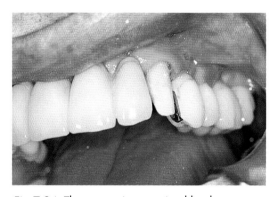

Fig 7.34 The restorations retained by the EsthetiCone abutments were screwed in place.

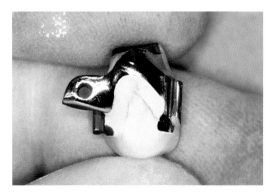

Fig 7.35 The canine crown was dried and made ready for final cementation after being tried in.

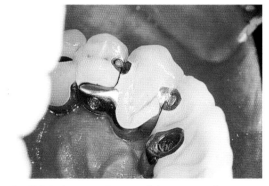

Fig 7.36 A mirror image of the crown after cementation showing the screw fully seated in the threaded tube in 12 and the interlocks similarly seated.

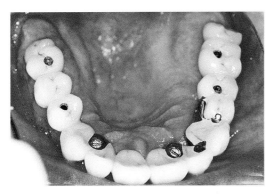

Fig 7.37 An occlusal view of the completed restorations after final tightening of the gold screws and cementation of the crown.

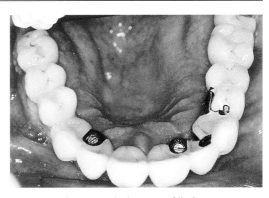

Fig 7.38 The screw holes were filled.

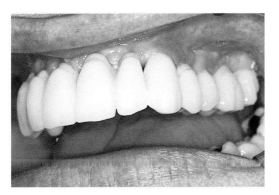

Fig 7.39 A buccal view of the left side.

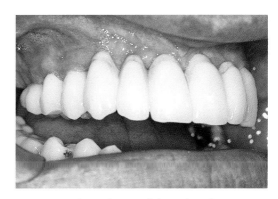

Fig 7.40 A buccal view of the right side.

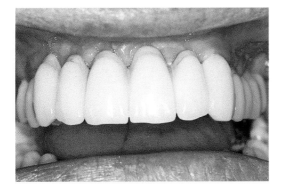

Fig 7.41 A buccal view of the anteriors.

The final stage was to fill the apertures through which the gold screws secured the restorations (Fig 7.38). Figures 7.39 to 7.41 show the completed case.

Case 2

An interesting situation is the case shown in Fig 7.42, where a patient had such an aversion to dentures that he tolerated the loss of all teeth in the maxillary left quadrant, with the exception of a single molar, without wearing one. The only attempt to replace the missing teeth

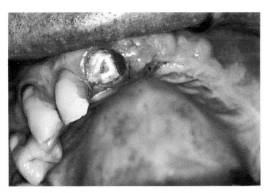

Fig 7.42 This patient presented with a direct cantilevered fixed partial denture replacing 9 which had fractured off the 8 abutment at gum level.

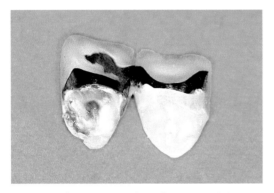

Fig 7.43 The direct cantilever fixed partial denture with the fractured abutment within the crown.

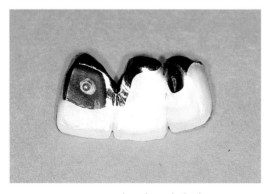

Fig 7.44 A pontic, with a threaded tube in the palatal surface, directly cantilevered from 7 and 8.

was a direct cantilever fixed partial denture (fitted by his previous dental surgeon) from the maxillary right central incisor, replacing the maxillary left central incisor. Unfortunately the right central incisor fractured at gum level, precipitating the need to address the problem of the missing teeth (Fig 7.43).

Three implants were placed at 10, 11 and 12. It was not possible to place implants at 9 or 13, 14 due to the presence, respectively, of a large incisive foramen and sinus in these areas. It was necessary, due to the bony anatomy, to correct angulation of the implants as esthetically as possible while providing retrievability. The three implants allowed a common path of withdrawal from a substructure built on three EsthetiCone abutments.

The maxillary left central incisor was replaced by a cantilever fixed partial denture, using the maxillary right central and lateral incisors as abutments (Fig 7.44). Forces on these abutments were reduced by the design of the completed restoration of the maxillary left quadrant.

Incorporated in the pontic was the tube section of the screw and tube precision attachment. A single tube was also incorporated in the subframe (Figs 7.45 and 7.46). The technician placed the tube so as to allow easy access to insert the screw. It can be seen in Figs 7.45 and 7.46 that the crown constructed on the molar has a cantilevered block which also houses a tube positioned horizontally and toward the mesial.

The subframe was shaped to provide a retentive form and also a natural-looking final contour for the superstructure. Lingual and buccal views, and one of the

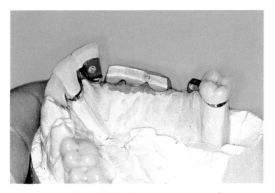

Fig 7.45 A threaded tube was positioned lingually in the 11, 12 region. The molar crown also had a threaded tube in the palatal surface of a cantilevered block extending mesially from it.

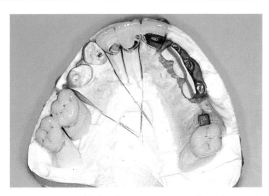

Fig 7.46 A milled substructure was placed on the implants.

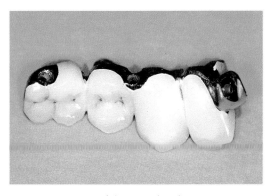

Fig 7.47 A view of the completed superstructure in which the apertures for the screws are clearly seen.

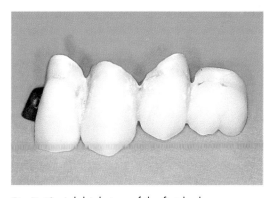

Fig 7.48 A labial view of the finished superstructure.

fitting surface, are shown in Figs 7.47 to 7.49. Projecting forwards from the lateral incisor is a 'wing' which overlaps the left central incisor pontic. When placed over the substructure retention is by means of the three screws only (Fig 7.50).

At the final appointment, having checked everything is fitting correctly, the molar crown and anterior fixed partial denture could be cemented (Figs 7.51 and 7.52). The superstructure was

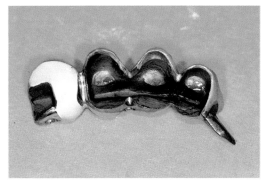

Fig 7.49 The fitting surface of the superstructure.

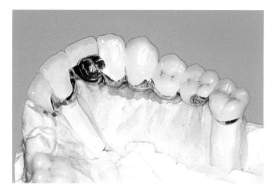

Fig 7.50 The fixed partial denture extending from 10 to 15 fully assembled on the working model.

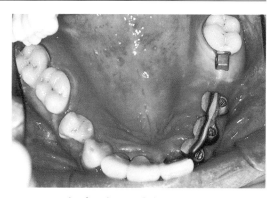

Fig 7.51 The fixed partial denture and the crown were cemented and the substructure screwed down fully.

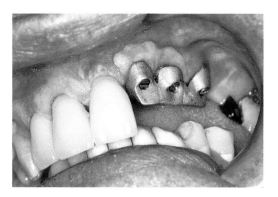

Fig 7.52 A labial view.

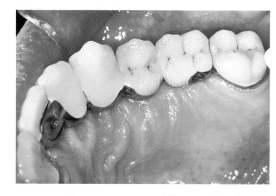

Fig 7.53 The superstructure fully seated and secured lingually by the three screws.

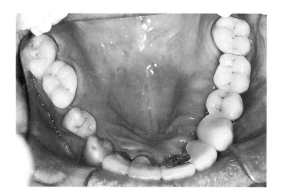

Fig 7.54 An occlusal view of the completed partial denture.

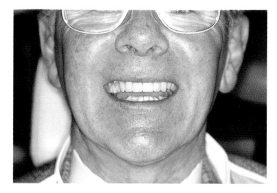

Fig 7.55 A happy patient.

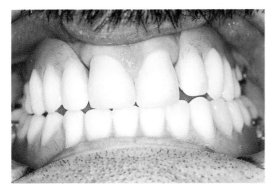

Fig 7.56 The appearance of the patient's mouth when presenting for treatment.

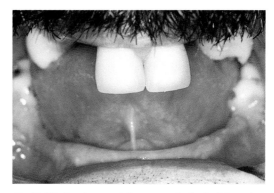

Fig 7.57 Teeth remaining were 2, 8, 9, 15 and 18, 31.

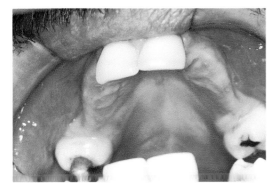

Fig 7.58 An occlusal view of the narrow maxillary arch.

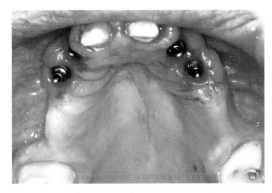

Fig 7.59 EsthetiCone abutments were placed on implants anterior to the sinuses.

then screwed into position (Fig 7.53). A semipermanent cement can be used but it is important that the screws are placed before this sets as clearing it out of the tubes can be difficult. Figures 7.54 and 7.55 show the final appearance.

Case 3

A patient with four maxillary and two mandibular teeth remaining at 2, 8, 9, 15 and 18, 31 requested implants and fixed partial dentures. Figures 7.56 to 7.58 show the pretreatment position. The maxillary arch was very narrow in relation to the

mandibular arch, resulting in a crossbite.

After careful case assessment, Nobel-Biocare implants were placed in the maxillary lateral incisor and canine positions on both sides of the arch and five similar implants in the symphysis of the mandibular arch. These, with the remaining teeth and suitable precision attachments, enabled the provision of a full-mouth oral rehabilitation with contingency for the removal of most units by the dentist. Six months later healing abutments were placed on these fixtures, followed by EsthetiCone abutments (Figs

105

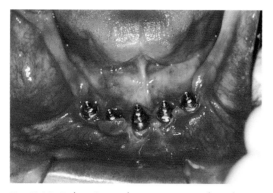

Fig 7.60 EsthetiCone abutments were placed on implants in the symphysis.

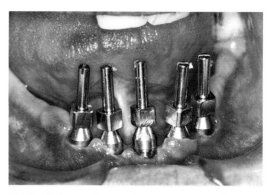

Fig 7.61 Impression copings were screwed onto the EsthetiCone abutments.

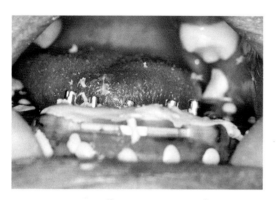

Fig 7.62 An overall impression was taken.

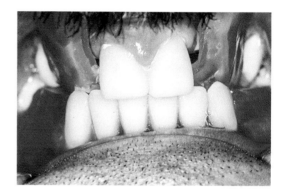

Fig 7.63 Getting the correct position of the mandibular anteriors.

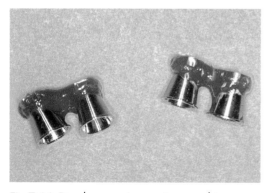

Fig 7.64 Duralay securing copings used to confirm the correct alignment of the analogues in the working model.

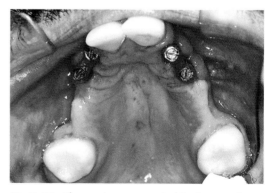

Fig 7.65. The copings were tried in the mouth.

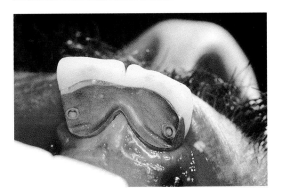

Fig 7.66 The maxillary central incisors were splinted together and threaded tubes were placed on their distolingual aspects.

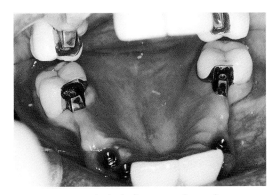

Fig 7.67 Extended platforms on the molars housed larger tubes.

7.59 and 7.60). An impression of each arch was taken, after preparation of the remaining teeth for full crowns using the screwblock technique (Figs 7.61 and 7.62).

A face-bow record was taken, as were centric, protrusive and lateral records. Temporary healing caps were placed on each of the abutments.

The next stage was to try in the mandibular teeth in wax (Fig 7.63) so that the technician would have a guide to the correct labiolingual positioning of the metal substructure. The accuracy of the working model can also be checked at this stage by placing copings over the analogues on the model and securing them in relation to each other using Palavit G or Duralay (Fig 7.64). These can be screwed gently into position in the mouth (Fig 7.65). Any malalignment shows up radiographic-ally: in this event a new impression must be taken before the next stage, the construction of the metal subframe.

When it was ready the subframe was tried in the patient's mouth, and then returned to the laboratory so that

the ceramic work could be completed.

In the maxillary arch both central incisors were splinted and the tubes from the screw and tube precision attachment housed within the framework on the distolingual aspects (Fig 7.66). Extended platforms from the molars housed larger tubes (Fig 7.67).

Two removable sections were then constructed over the implants with extended anterior wings which passed over the lingual aspect of the framework on the incisors, and a superstructure which fitted distally over the extended platforms off the molars. Both sections had an aperture at each end, through which a screw secured the fixed partial denture to the incisors and molar on each side. Gold screws were also used to secure the fixed partial dentures to the fixtures (Figs 7.68 to 7.70).

In the mandibular arch five fixtures secured the six mandibular anterior teeth with the matrix for a Roach attachment at the distal of each canine (Figs 7.71 and 7.72). Again, the molars had extended platforms housing a tube.

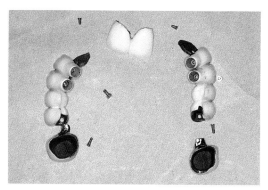

Fig 7.68 The fitting surfaces of the crowns and removable fixed partial dentures for the maxillary arch.

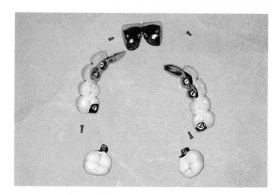

Fig 7.69 The occlusal surfaces of the crowns and removable fixed partial dentures.

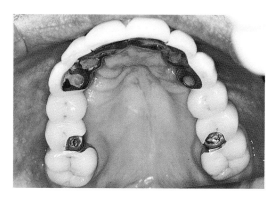

Fig 7.70 The completed maxillary arch giving easy access to the implants if required.

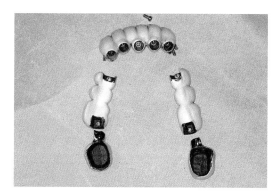

Fig 7.71 The crowns and removable fixed partial dentures for the mandibular arch.

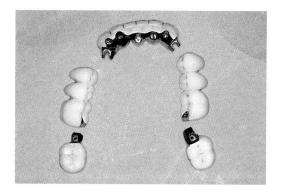

Fig 7.72 An occlusal view of the component parts for the mandibular arch.

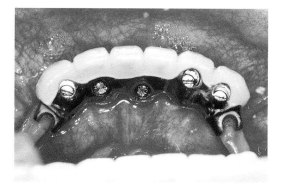

Fig 7.73 A close-up view of the Roach attachment matrices in the mandibular arch.

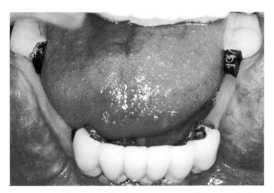

Fig 7.74 The mandibular crowns with extended platforms containing threaded tubes.

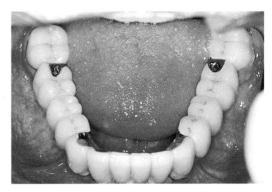

Fig 7.75. The mandibular removable fixed partial dentures fitted and allowing flexion of the mandible without stressing the ceramometal reconstruction.

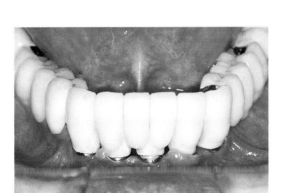

Fig 7.76 Spaces between the restorations allowed easy access for cleaning.

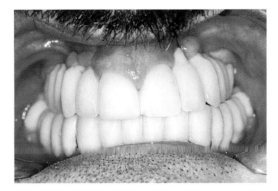

Fig 7.77 The maxillary and mandibular arches in occlusion.

The third section for each side was a removable partial denture which allowed the passage of a screw to secure it within the tube in the extended platform distally, while the patrix of the Roach attachment was housed mesially.

Figures 7.73 to 7.75 show the final stages of fitting for the mandibular arch, Fig 7.76 the spaces that will allow good hygiene around the implant, and Figs 7.77 and 7.78 the completed work.

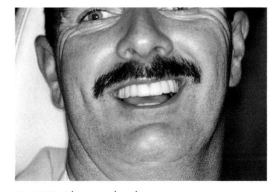

Fig 7.78 The completed case.

The design in the last case allows for the removal in the maxillary arch of eight units. This provides easy access to the implants and their abutments for inspection and maintenance. Any fracture repair would also be facilitated.

In the mandibular arch the splinted crowns on the five fixtures provide a very rigid unit anteriorly. Hobkirk et al[5] raised concern over the rigid connection of implants between the symphysis of the mandible and the posterior mandible. Burch[6] also found that the magnitude of mandibular flexion increased distal to the metal foramen.

The Roach attachments in the first premolar positions allow some movement to take place, which compensates for the inherent flexibility of the mandible. It also allows fixed partial dentures to be provided that extend from the second molars to the canines without the need for more implant support distally.

Short Cantilever Fixed Partial Dentures and Overdentures

There follows a discussion of an alternative treatment to short cantilever fixed partial dentures and overdentures. The next two cases do not involve the use of teeth in combination with implants but they are included here as the author has found them particularly useful.

If short implants are placed in the anterior part of the mandible in a very shallow curvature, it is unwise to cantilever more than a single unit distally as

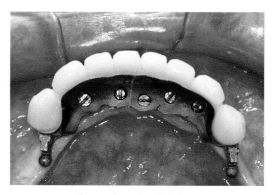

Fig 7.79 Implants placed with little antero-posterior spread limited the distal cantilever. In this case a single unit was cantilevered distally and Dalbo precision attachments were connected distally.

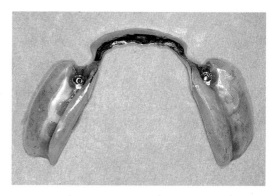

Fig 7.80 The precision attachment-retained mandibular partial denture.

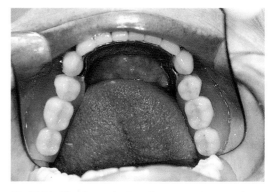

Fig 7.81 The lingual plate fitting neatly over the metal framework of the fixed partial denture.

stresses would be transferred to the screws and fixtures.[4] The design in the following case allows for a complete restoration of the mandibular arch.

Case 4

Figure 7.79 shows five implants supporting an anterior fixed partial denture. The first premolars have been cantilevered distally and carry precision attachments that help to stressbreak occlusal forces on the fixed partial denture. The attachment used was the Dalbo-S resilient joint, which allows both a hinge and vertical movement.

Figure 7.80 shows the matrix housed in the mandibular denture and Fig 7.81 is an occlusal view of it. This design ensures that the patient has good function posteriorly and excellent stability of the mandibular denture: the anterior fixed partial denture provides support and retention without excessive loading of the implants and associated structures. Figures 7.82 to 7.84 show the completed work.

Case 5

In the maxillary arch there are greater restrictions on the provision of implant supported fixed partial dentures. The quality of the bone is not generally as good. The ridges are often thinner than ideal, restricting the diameter of implants, and the sinuses, which are frequently pneumatized, extend forwards and downwards, close to the canines, limiting their placement to the anterior segment.

Conventional treatments for such patients provided fixed partial dentures or overdentures. For fixed partial dentures the extent of the cantilever distally would depend on the length and

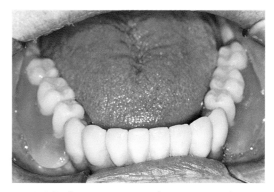

Fig 7.82 The precision attachment-retained denture sits securely and fully restores the posterior quadrants.

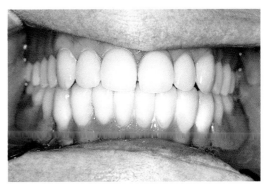

Fig 7.83 The maxillary and mandibular arches in occlusion.

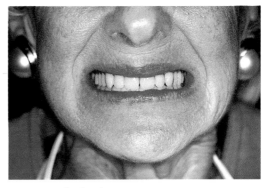

Fig 7.84 The final appearance.

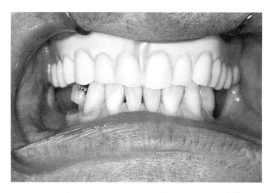

Fig 7.85 The patient presented wearing a full maxillary denture and with missing posterior teeth.

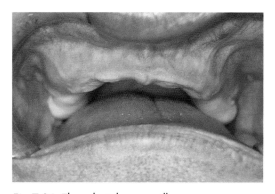

Fig 7.86 The edentulous maxilla.

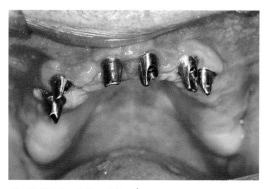

Fig 7.87 Steri-Oss DIA abutments.

diameter of the fixtures and on the forces opposing the restoration. Inevitably in such situations the distance cantilevered is often compromised, with fixed partial dentures extending no further than the first or second premolars, leaving the molar areas unrestored.

My own experience over the past eight years convinces me that there is a better option for the many patients in this category. Sinus augmentation is one solution. However, as many patients baulk at this procedure, I have found a way around the common problem, a treatment which can be applied to dentate patients and which is frequently used by me and others working with precision attachments.

The treatment involves the use of the maxillary anterior teeth to retain a precision attachment-retained denture replacing teeth in the posterior quadrants. Even when teeth have lost bony support they can be splinted together to retain a denture. Stress-breakage is provided where necessary by an attachment such as the Dalbo which has not only a hinge movement but also vertical displacement, resisted under loading by a spring housed within the matrix. If the degree of stress-breakage needed is less, then the PR attachment is suitable.

I have used this treatment on patients with an edentulous maxillary arch to provide fixed anterior partial dentures combined with the restoration of the posterior quadrants with a precision attachment-retained prosthesis. Acceptance by patients is high as they feel this is superior to the provision of an overdenture. Though it provides one premolar less than fixed partial dentures, there is

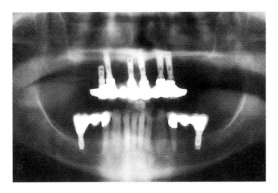

Fig 7.88 A radiograph showing that the placement of implants in the premaxilla was limited by the pneumatized maxillary sinuses.

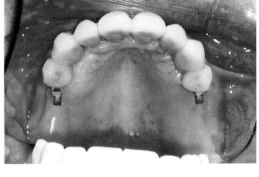

Fig 7.89 The distally cantilevered pontics 5, 12 had PR attachments connected to them.

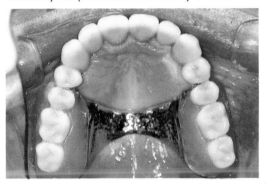

Fig 7.90 The denture securely seated and restoring good function and esthetics in the posterior quadrants.

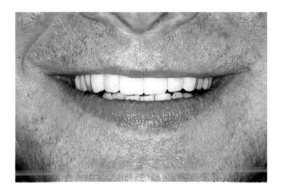

Fig 7.91 The final appearance.

a complete restoration of the arch. It is necessary to reduce one premolar unit in order to attach the patrices of the attachments within the stress distribution limits. The advantages are better esthetics and function for little extra cost.

Figures 7.85 and 7.86 are preoperative views of a patient who had large maxillary sinuses that extended forward to the canine region and left only one or two millimetres of bone beneath the sinuses in the posterior segments. The ridges anteriorly varied in thickness and height

allowing implants to be placed which were long (with one exception) but varied in diameter between narrow and regular. The abutments are shown in Fig 7.87 and a radiograph (Fig 7.88) shows the fixed partial denture and attachments as well as the large maxillary sinuses.

The splinted crowns on the abutments with the cantilevered premolar pontics and PR attachments can be seen in Fig 7.89. The precision attachment-retained maxillary denture fits securely into these (Figs 7.90 and 7.91).

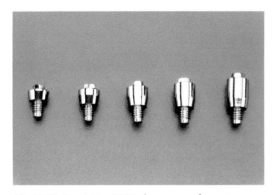

Fig 7.92 Steri-Oss PME abutments of varying length.

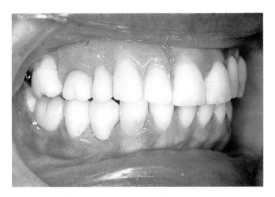

Fig 7.93 The patient presented wearing an acrylic denture replacing 3 to 7, 10 and 13.

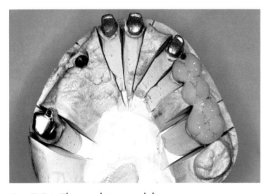

Fig 7.94 The working model.

PME Abutments

The PME abutment (Fig 7.92) comes in lengths of 2, 3, 4, 5 and 6 mm. It is made of titanium alloy and is capable of as much as a 40° misalignment correction between implants. This versatility makes it useful for fixed-removable restorations.

Applications of the PME Steri-Oss abutment are:

- Fixed-removable full arch reconstructions on six or more attachments.
- Overdentures supported on implants attached to a bar on four to six implants.
- Tissue supported overdentures attached to a bar on two implants.
- Fixed-removable partial denture on two or more implants.
- Fixed-removable partial denture attached to natural teeth with precision attachments.

The discussion here will be limited to an example of the last application.

Case 6

Precision attachments were used with the PME abutment to provide contingency planning as well as splinting and distribution of lateral forces for the patient shown in Fig 7.93. Here a maxillary acrylic denture with full palatal coverage replaced 3 to 7, 10 and 13.

The implant was placed in the 6 position owing to the availability of bone in that region. After exposure six months later (following confirmation of integration) the PME abutment was screwed into the implant. An impression coping was screwed onto the abutment and an overall impression was taken in silicone. The coping was then removed and relocalized into the impression. A temporary healing cap was placed over the abutment.

Figure 7.94 is the working model with a fixed partial denture extending from 12 to 14 which had a Stern Tube-lock precision attachment placed mesially in the first premolar to give additional support to the anterior fixed partial denture. 2 had an inner gold thimble with screw and tube mesially. Figure 7.95 shows this in the mouth.

The anterior fixed partial denture extended from the maxillary left canine to the right lateral incisor. There was a screw and tube in the pontic at 7, as well as a pinhole (Fig 7.96).

A fixed partial denture was also constructed to replace 3 and 4. A crown was placed as a retainer on 2 and the metal substructure of the partial denture was extended forwards over the implant analogue, to which it was secured by means of the coping screw (Fig 7.97).

This metal extension over the implants was designed with the labial surface cut back and the height of the coping screw reduced so that a countersink provided additional retention for an overlying crown. The screw was cut down with a Carborundum disc and a new screwdriver slot cut into the end of it with the edge of the disc.

A Stern Tube-lock precision attachment was placed in the mesial of the 4 pontic. It had a path of withdrawal identical to the substructure over the implant analogue and to the pinhole in 7.

A crown was then made to fit over the

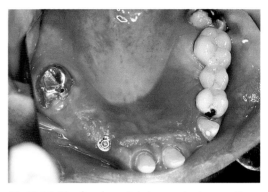

Fig 7.95 The fixed partial denture in the maxillary left quadrant carries an interlock matrix mesially in 12. A PME abutment is seen at 6 and an inner gold thimble with threaded tube mesially in 2.

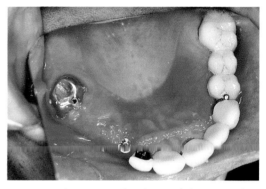

Fig 7.96 The anterior fixed partial denture with interlock patrix and cantilevered pontic at 7.

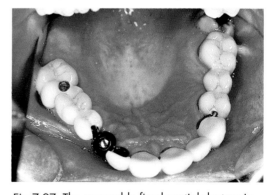

Fig 7.97 The removable fixed partial denture in the maxillary right quadrant, screwed onto the 2 thimble distally and into the PME abutment mesially. 4 had a Stern Tube-lock matrix mesially.

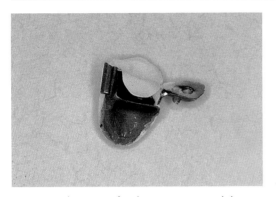

Fig 7.98 The crown for the canine carried the patrix of a Stern Tube-lock distally, and a cantilevered wing containing the collar of the screw and tube precision attachment, as well as a pin.

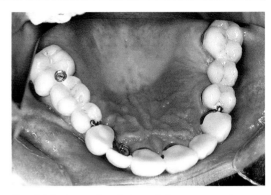

Fig 7.99 An occlusal view of the connected crown and fixed partial dentures in the maxillary arch.

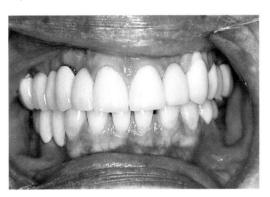

Fig 7.100 Centric occlusion.

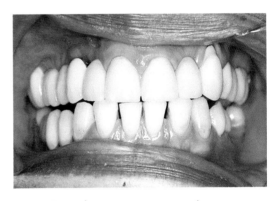

Fig 7.101 Balance in protrusive occlusion.

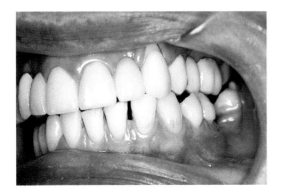

Fig 7.102 Left lateral excursion.

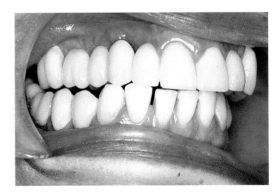

Fig 7.103 Right lateral excursion.

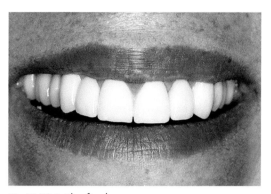

Fig 7.104 The final appearance.

substructure incorporating the patrix of the Stern Tube-lock, as well as the mesial extension over the 7 pontic. This extension contained the collar for the screw and tube precision attachment, and also a pin (Fig 7.98). Figure 7.99 shows the occlusal view of the completed work.

Figure 7.100 shows centric occlusion, Fig 7.101 protrusive occlusion and Figs 7.102 and 7.103 lateral excursion, while Fig 7.104 is a labial view.

The treatment described above has the following advantages:

· The use of precision attachments means that the implant at 6 can be splinted effectively to the adjacent natural teeth, reducing the loading on it, especially in lateral excursion.
· The number of implants required to support the fixed partial denture can be reduced, thus saving the patient greater surgical trauma.
· The cost to the patient is thus also reduced; for many this is a major consideration.
· In the event of failure, the whole super-

structure distal to the 7 pontic can be unscrewed for repair or to allow further treatment to the implant.
· Esthetics are improved by this dentist-removable partial denture.

Interlocks

Interlocks are extremely useful in restorative dentistry as they allow a degree of both splinting and retrievability. They are also relatively inexpensive.

When they are used to splint a tooth or teeth to an implant or implants it is important that a careful assessment is made of the extent of the force on the implant retained restoration. If it is felt that this could prejudice the success of the implant then the clinician would be wiser to avoid such a plan. It is necessary to consider the extent and direction of the added force, the length and diameter of the implant, the quality of the bone and the angulation of the implants in that bone.

Case 7

Figure 7.105 shows a case where a molar which had previously been the distal abutment of a failed fixed partial denture, and which had also lost a little bony support, stood alone in the maxillary left quadrant, the only posterior tooth remaining distal to the canine. Because of the loss of bone it was decided that the tooth should not be used as a fixed partial denture abutment. Fortunately the previous dentist had inserted a mesial interlock which could be used to splint the molar to the two implants.

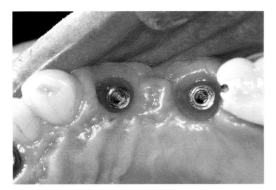

Fig 7.105 Implants were placed at 12 and 14. 15 had lost a little bony support and an interlock matrix remained in the mesial of the crown.

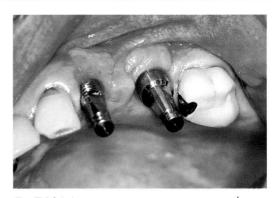

Fig 7.106 Impression copings were screwed onto the fixture heads.

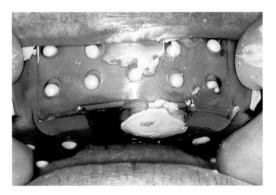

Fig 7.107 An accurate overall impression was taken.

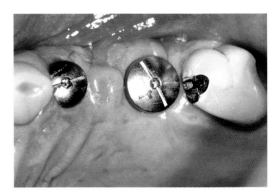

Fig 7.108 Healing abutments were replaced on the fixtures.

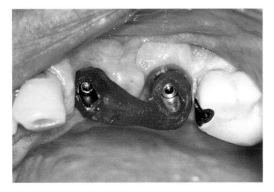

Fig 7.109 The Steri-Oss abutments were positioned on the implant heads using a Duralay jig.

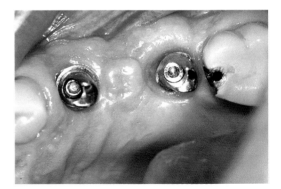

Fig 7.110 The Duralay jig was removed.

Two Steri-Oss impression copings were placed on the fixtures (Fig 7.106). A plastic patrix for a Stern Tube-lock was placed in the matrix within the crown leaving an extension of approximately 5 to 6 mm projecting beyond the occlusal surface. This will provide stability for the patrix when the overall impression is taken (Fig 7.107).

The impression copings were unscrewed and dispatched to the laboratory with the impressions, a centric record and face-bow recording. The healing abutments were then replaced (Fig 7.108).

DIA Steri-Oss abutments were modelled by the technician in the laboratory before construction of the metal substructure, incorporating the interlock in the molar which would help stabilize the tooth.

To help localize the DIA abutments accurately on the fixture, the technician constructed an acrylic resin jig with apertures to allow the passage of the abutment screws (Fig 7.109). This was then removed from the mouth (Fig 7.110) and the metal substructure tried in. It should fit passively and accurately (Fig 7.111). When this was confirmed it could be removed from the mouth, together with the DIA abutments.

If there had been a problem with the fit of the metal substructure then this would have been sectioned and relocalized and the fit rechecked before proceeding.

The final stage was the replacement of the abutments on the fixtures (Figs 7.112 to 7.114) using the Steri-Oss torque wrench (which delivers 35 NCM torque)

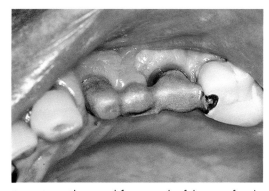

Fig 7.111 The metal framework of the new fixed partial denture was placed on the abutments. The patrix of the interlock attached distally to the framework is seated fully into the matrix in 15.

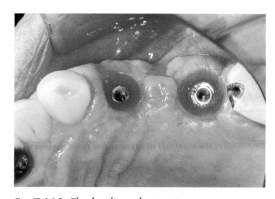

Fig 7.112 The healing abutments were removed prior to the final fitting of the fixed partial denture.

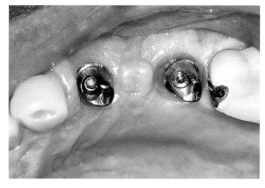

Fig 7.113 The abutments replaced on the fixture heads.

119

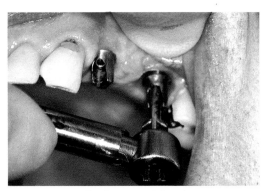

Fig 7.114 Final tightening of the abutment screws using a torque wrench.

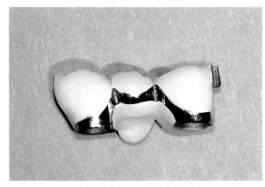

Fig 7.115 A lingual view of the fixed partial denture.

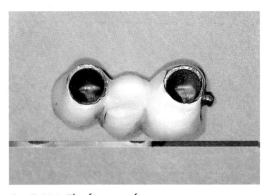

Fig 7.116 The fitting surface.

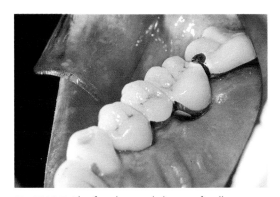

Fig 7.117 The fixed partial denture finally cemented.

for final tightening of the abutment screws.

Figures 7.115 and 7.116 are views of the lingual and fitting surfaces of the final restoration. Figure 7.117 is of the restoration after final cementation in the mouth. The case which follows also involves the use of interlocks.

Patients are sometimes loathe to lose teeth even when extraction might be beneficial. There are of course situations where it is advantageous to retain teeth

for both clinical and psychological reasons. If they are well sited they can be used to help position implants correctly. Stents placed on these teeth can be extremely helpful in this regard. Another advantage of retaining teeth is that proprioception is not lost provided the teeth have some freedom of movement.

Case 8

Figure 7.118 is a computed tomographic view of a case where a patient had four

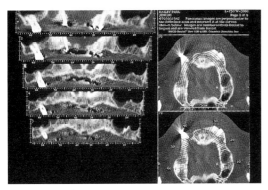

Fig 7.118 The CT scan.

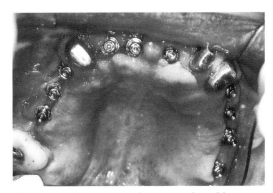

Fig 7.119 EsthetiCone abutments placed between the remaining teeth.

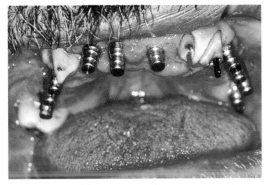

Fig 7.120 Gold copings on the anterior teeth were removed and the teeth were prepared for crowns. Impression copings were placed on the abutments ready for an overall impression to be taken.

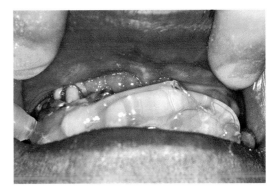

Fig 7.121 The copings could help to provide an initial occlusal record for the technician.

maxillary teeth remaining: the maxillary right second molar and canine and the maxillary left lateral incisor and canine. The maxillary right canine had also drifted distally. All the maxillary anterior teeth had previously been root filled and they had had gold copings placed. A partial overdenture had been worn over these.

Ten implants were placed and Estheti-Cone abutments screwed down onto them (Fig 7.119). Impression copings were screwed onto these and an overall impression was taken which included the preparations on the anterior teeth (Fig 7.120). Provided the patient can close in centric relation at the correct vertical dimension these impression copings can be useful as they help to provide an initial occlusal record for the technician (Fig 7.121).

An accurate record was taken prior to construction of the metalwork. From this record a wax try-in of the teeth was

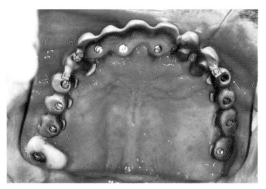

Fig 7.122 The metal framework was tried in with Stern Tube-lock matrices both mesially and distally on 6, mesially on 10, and distally on 11.

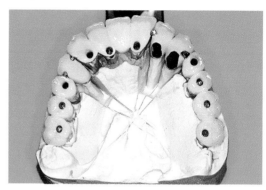

Fig 7.123 The crown and fixed partial dentures were fully assembled on the working model.

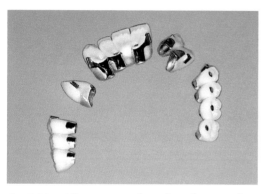

Fig 7.124 All units apart from those housing the matrices were splinted together.

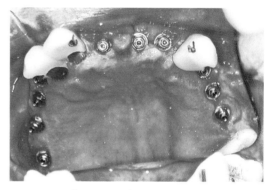

Fig 7.125 The crowns housing the matrices were cemented. The lateral incisor and canine were splinted to reduce stress on the posts.

provided. When this was found to be acceptable it could then be used to provide matrix keys of the labial and buccal surfaces which would allow the correct positioning of the metal sub-structure.

Figure 7.122 shows the metalwork at the try-in stage, when it was found to fit passively and accurately. The matrices of the interlocks were placed in the crowns on the anterior teeth; the

maxillary right canine had one placed mesially and distally. The maxillary left lateral and canine were splinted and the attachments were fitted in the mesial of the lateral and the distal of the canine. The patrices were placed on the crowns on the adjacent EsthetiCone abutments.

In this case the bases of the matrices were cut away allowing complete freedom of movement between them and

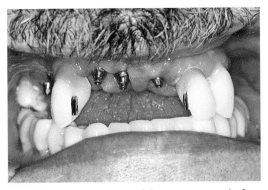

Fig 7.126 A labial view of the matrices and of the pink porcelain used cervically to reduce the apparent length of the crowns.

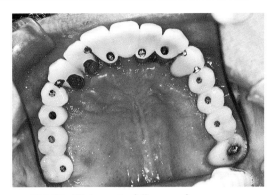

Fig 7.127 All the units fully seated.

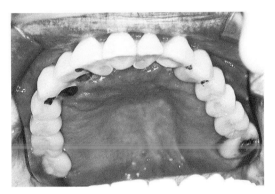

Fig 7.128 The gold screw apertures were filled with composite resin.

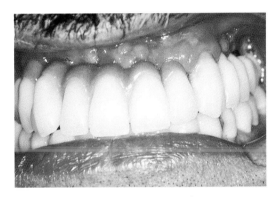

Fig 7.129 Pink porcelain was used on anterior units to mimic soft tissue.

the patrices. In this way the splinted crowns on the implants could be removed without disturbing those on the natural teeth and the converse was equally true — it would be possible for the crowns on the natural teeth to be removed without affecting the splinted implant crowns.

The next stage was the application of the porcelain in the laboratory (Figs 7.123 and 7.124).

Figures 7.125 and 7.126 show the crowns cemented on the natural teeth. Figure 7.127 shows the implant crowns after they were secured on the abutments by means of gold screws. Figure 7.128 is an occlusal view of the completed arch. Pink porcelain was used anteriorly to mimic the lost soft and hard tissue (Fig 7.129).

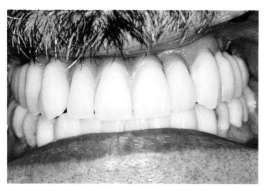

Fig 7.130 Centric occlusion anteriorly.

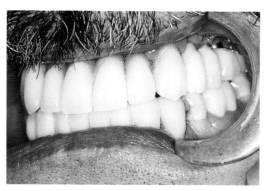

Fig 7.131 Centric occlusion on the left side.

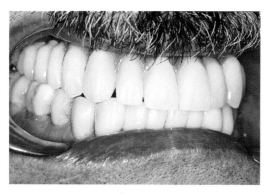

Fig 7.132 Centric occlusion on the right side.

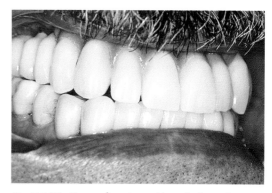

Fig 7.133 Group function with right lateral excursion.

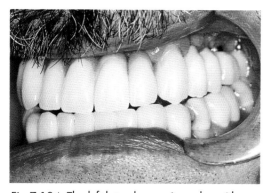

Fig 7.134 The left lateral excursion, also with group function.

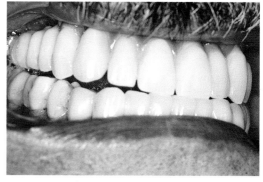

Fig 7.135 Balance in protrusive movement of the mandible.

The Importance of Checking Occlusion

In a case such as this it is imperative that great care is taken to balance the occlusion. This means applying all the basic principles of occlusion. Failure to do this will overload the teeth, the implants or the component parts of the implants and superstructure.

Figures 7.130 to 7.132 show centric occlusion anteriorly, and on both the left and right sides. Figure 7.133 shows the right lateral excursion and a group function to reduce lateral forces, Fig 7.134 the left lateral excursion with a group function. Figure 7.135 is a view showing balance in protrusive movement of the mandible.

References

1 *Lindquist LW; Rockler B; Carlsson GE.* Bone resorption around fixtures in edentulous patients treated with mandibular fixed tissue-integrated prostheses. J Prosthet Dent 59: 50-63, 1988.

2 *Lekholm U.* Clinical procedures for treatment with osseointegrated dental implants. J Prosthet Dent 50: 116-120, 1983.

3 *Langer B; Sullivan DY.* Osseointegration: Its impact on the inter-relationship of periodontics and restorative dentistry: Part II. Int J Periodont Rest Dent 9: 165-183, 1989.

4 *Rangert B; Jemt T Jörneus L.* Forces and movements on Brånemark implants. Int J Oral Maxillofac Implants. Vol 4, No 3, 1989.

5 *Hobkirk JA; Schwab J.* Mandibular deformation in subjects with osseointegrated implants. Int J Oral Maxillofac Implants 6: 319-328, 1991.

6 *Burch JG.* The dynamic mandibular arch width. In: Lurdeen HC; Gibbs CH (eds). Advances in Occlusion 81-87. Boston: John Wright PSG Inc, 1982.

Further Reading

Brånemark P-I; Zarb GA; Albrektsson T. Tissue-Integrated Prostheses. Chicago: Quintessence Publishing Co, 1985.

The EsthetiCone: An abutment alternative for esthetic implant restorations. J Esthet Dent Update. Vol 2, No 2, April 1991.

Ganne J; Astrad P; Ahten K; Borg K; Olsson M. Implants in partially edentulous patients: A longitudinal study of bridges supported by both implants and natural teeth. Clinical Oral Implant Res 3: 49-56, 1992.

Hobo S; Ichida E; Goresia LT. Osseointegration and Occlusal Rehabilitation. Chicago: Quintessence Publishing Co, 1990.

Parel SM. The Smiline™ System. Dallas, Texas: Taylor Publishing Co.

Rangert B; Gunne J; Sullivan DY. Mechanical aspects of a Brånemark implant connected to a natural tooth: An in vitro study. Int J Oral Maxillofac Implants 6: 177-186, 1991.

Rieder CE. Copings on tooth and implant abutments for superstructure prostheses. Int J Periodont Rest Dent 10: 437-453, 1990.

Appendix

Extracoronal Precision Attachments

Extracoronal attachments can be rigid but are generally resilient, distributing the potentially harmful forces away from the abutments to the edentulous ridges. This is especially useful with free-end saddles.

The patrix of extracoronal attachments is either soldered or cast to the retainer adjoining a saddle area and is completely outside the normal contour of that retainer. The matrix is housed within the prosthesis.

Extracoronal Rigid Slide Attachments

1. Bi-Nat. MP
Height 4 mm
In the case of bilateral or unilateral free-end saddles, a hinge arm can be attached to the patrix, which will allow the saddle to move towards the ridge independently of the metal framework.
Application Bilateral free-end saddles, operator removable fixed partial dentures, and partial dentures.
Activation There is a synthetic friction buffer housed in the patrix. Turn the locking screw to expand the synthetic friction buffer and increase the retention. Alternatively, replace the friction buffer.

2. *Conex Slide Attachment. CM
Height 5 mm
Application Fixed or operator removable partial dentures and implant suprastructures. Rigid unilateral free-end dentures transversely locked and rigid bilateral free-end dentures.
Activation To increase friction, spread the lamellae of the cone with activator.

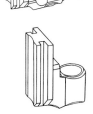

---

*These attachments are adjustable and require rigid bracing support to protect them against leverage forces which could reduce the retention between matrix and patrix. The lingual or palatal walls of the retainer pontic are milled parallel to the path of insertion of the attachments, with a groove milled in the opposite approximal surface from the attachment. A bracing arm is waxed up, cast, and soldered to the attachment which will be housed in the removable prosthesis. The cervical finishing line of the bracing arm should be lower than the attachment.

3. Flecher Screw-retained Slide Attachment. CM

Height 4 mm
Application Fixed or operator-removable partial dentures and implant supra- structures. Partial

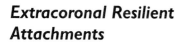

dentures with operator-removable bars with screw-retained connections to crowns.

Extracoronal Resilient Attachments

1. Dalbo-S Resilient Joint. CM

Height 5 mm (matrix)
Application To retain unilateral and bilateral free-end dentures. Long denture saddles with transversal bar. Vertical

translation and rotational movements. When used in a unilateral case, cross-arch stabilization must be used to protect the attachment.
Activation Bend lamellae of the matrix towards the centre with an instrument.

2. Mini-Dalbo Hinge by Dr Dalla Bona. CM

Height 3 mm (matrix)
Application To retain unilateral and bilateral free-end saddle dentures.

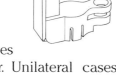

Short and long saddles with transversal bar. Unilateral cases require cross-arch stabilization.
Activation the same as that described for Dalbo-S.

3. Hinge by Roach. CM

Height 4.8 mm; can be shortened by 1.2 mm
Application Hinged unilateral and bilateral free-end saddles.

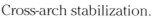
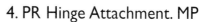

Cross-arch stabilization.
Activation Activate the patrix with a scalpel or activating tool.

4. PR Hinge Attachment. MP

Height 4.5 mm
Application
Unilateral and bilateral free-end partial dentures.
The PR hinge eliminates undesirable lateral

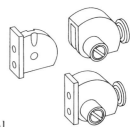

movement which makes it possible in the unilateral free-end saddle situation to dispense with cross-arch stabilization in some cases.
Activation To increase retention, screw in the locking screw which is housed in the matrix, or replace the plastic cushion and plunger.

5. *Ceka Revax Extracoronal Attachment

There are four different matrices available. The angles of the matrix arms are 15, 30, 45, or 60 degrees. The greater the angle, the larger the embrasure between the matrix and the retainer.

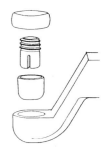

There are two types of matrix keeper: (a) a precision matrix fixed in the keeper with a special bonding composite; (b) a precision matrix incorporated in a burn-out plastic pattern and cast onto. The patrix pin can be screwed into three types of retentive elements to retain the attachment in the denture (the spacer technique, soldering, and acrylic resin retention). The attachment must have 5 mm clearance between the ridge adjacent to the abutment tooth and the opposing occlusal surface. It must have bracing support.

Application Removable free-end and bounded saddle partial dentures. Can be rigid or resilient.

Activation Spread the segments of the patrix with an activating tool.

Intracoronal Slide Attachments

Here the matrix is contained within the contour of the crown. For this the clinician will need to prepare boxes in order to accommodate the attachment. It is useful during the preparation to have either the attachment or a plastic dummy to help ensure that sufficient space is provided. To guarantee diffusion of the metal casting onto the attachment, it is necessary to enlarge the width and depth of the box by 0.6 to 0.2 mm in comparison with the actual size of the attachment. Before preparing the abutment, make sure it is possible to cut a box large enough to house

the matrix within the confines of the natural contour of the tooth.

There are two groups of intracoronal attachments: nonadjustable and adjustable. All are rigid.

Nonadjustable Intracoronal Attachments

1. Rod and Tube Attachment. MP

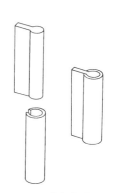

Application Fixed partial dentures with a minor alignment problem of the abutments. Used as a connector for dentures and to support one end of a removable partial denture which is retained at the other end by an adjustable retentive attachment.

2. Cylindrical Slide Attachment. CM

Application The same as that described for Rod and Tube Attachments.

3. Stern Tube-lock. APM-Sterngold

Patrix and matrix elements are plastic burn-out patterns which are incorporated into the wax patterns and cast.
Application The same as that described for Rod and Tube Attachments.

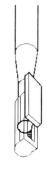

4. Preat-Contur

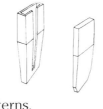

Slide attachment tapering from the occlusal surface to the cervical margin. Patrix and matrix elements are plastic burn-out patterns.

Application Minor alignment problems with nonparallel abutments and fixed-movable partial dentures.

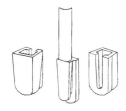

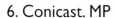

5. Preat Better Plastic Dovetail

Application The same as that de-scribed for Preat-Contur.

6. Conicast. MP

A tapered slide attachment with plastic burn-out patterns.
Application The same as that described for Preat-Contur.

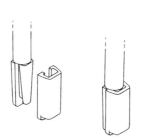

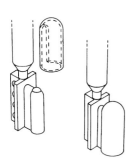

7. Intracast. MP

A slide attachment with plastic burn-out patterns.
Application The same as that de-scribed for Rod and Tube Attach-ments.

8. Omcast. MP

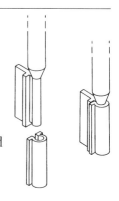

A slide attachment with plastic burn-out patterns.
Application
The same as that described for Rod and Tube Attachments.

9. Dovetail Slide Attachment by Professor Beyeler. CM

Application Posterior fixed partial dentures with minor alignment problem of the abutments, and as a connector.

10. Key and Keyway. Laboratory-made Attachment

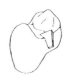

Application Used to correct minor alignment problems in fixed partial denture con-struction, and in fixed and semifixed dentures when minor and major retainers are used.

Adjustable Intracoronal Attachments

1. *Ancra. MP

Application Remov-able fixed partial dentures, cross-arch stabilization, partial dentures, and minor alignment problems with posterior abutment teeth.
Activation Expand the slot with a suit-able instrument.

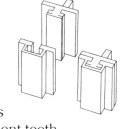

2. *T-123. MP

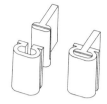

Application and Activation The same as that described for Ancra.

3. *McCollum. MP

The active side of the patrix must face buccally to allow activation without interference from the lingual or palatal bracing support.

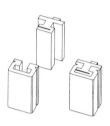

Application Fixed partial dentures, removable partial dentures, unilateral and bilateral free-end dentures and cross-arch stabilization. *Activation* Expand the slot with an instrument.

4. *McCollum T-shaped Slide Attachment. CM

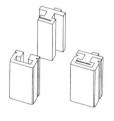

Application and Activation The same as that described for McCollum.

5. *Stern Gingival Latch. APM-Sterngold

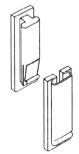

Application The same as that described for McCollum.
Activation Expand the slot at the base of the patrix with a special gauge.

Anchors

These attachments are used on either roots or implants to retain overdentures or removable partial dentures. The patrix is soldered to the diaphragm of a cast post and the matrix contained in the denture.

There are two basic types: rigid and resilient. The rigid attachments are used in bounded unilateral or bilateral saddle cases and the resilient attachments, which allow a degree of movement between the patrix and matrix, reducing the stress on the abutment roots, are used in bilateral free-end saddle cases. If used unilaterally to retain a removable partial denture, a transversal connector must be used to give cross-arch stabilization which will lessen the stress on the abutment tooth or teeth.

Rigid Anchors

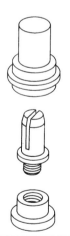

1. Introfix. MP

Height 4.7 mm
Application Can be used to retain partial dentures and removable fixed partial dentures. The Introfix must always be used in conjunction with one or more other attachments.

All attachments marked * when used to retain a removable partial denture must have rigid bracing support to protect the attachment from undue overloading. This is achieved by milling the lingual or palatal surfaces of the retainer and a cast secondary bracing arm attached to the denture. All cast metal denture frameworks must be completely rigid.

Activation Spreading the friction pin or replacing it with a new one.

2. Anchor by Dr Conod. CM

Height 3.5 mm
Application To retain rigid hybrid dentures.
Activation Spread the patrix with a scalpel or activator.

3. Eccentric Rothermann. CM

Height 1.1 mm
Application The same as that described for Anchor by Dr Conod. The patrix has a core of solder in the centre of the attachment which makes the soldering of

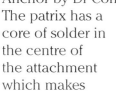

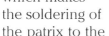

the patrix to the diaphragm a relatively simple operation.
Activation Bend the clasp arms of the matrix towards the centre.

4. Gerber-RZ 32.02 Retention Cylinder by Professor Gerber. CM

Height 4 mm
Application The same as that described for Anchor by Dr Conod. This attachment is multifunctional and therefore useful in contingency planning. The base of the patrix has a threaded post onto which is screwed a retentive core. This allows for conversion to other

types of anchor at a later stage, such as the Schubiger-SB 33.01 Screwblock, which has a height of 2.8 mm. If two or more are used with an adequate space between them, a bar can be soldered to the matrix sleeves and used to retain an overdenture. The Schubiger-SB

33.02 has a height of 7 mm and can be used to retain operator-removable crowns and partial dentures. The patrix of the Gerber-RZ 32.02 can also be converted to a resilient Dalbo-B 52089 and used to retain an overdenture.
Activation Replace the split ring in the matrix.

6. Schubiger-SB 33.02 Screwblock. CM

Height 7 mm
Application To retain operator-removable crowns and partial dentures as described for Gerber-RZ 32.02.

7. Ceka Axial Attachment. Ceka NV

Application To retain removable partial dentures and overdentures. The space maintainer is not used between the diaphragm and the fitting surface of the denture.
Activation Spread the segments of the patrix with an activating tool.

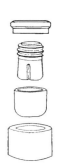

Resilient Anchors

1. Compact. MP

Height 2.85 mm
Application To retain overdentures.
Activation Bend lamellae of the matrix towards the centre.

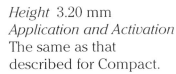

2. Profix. MP

Height 3.20 mm
Application and Activation The same as that described for Compact.

3. Eccentric Rothermann Resilient Anchor. CM

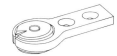

Height 1.7 mm
Application The same as that described for Compact.
Activation Bend the clasp arms of the matrix towards the centre.

4. Dalbo-Z Cylindrical Anchor. CM

Height 4 mm
Application and Activation The same as that described for Compact.

5. Supra-Snap. MP

Application There are various types of patrix which can be screwed into compatible implants to retain an overdenture.
Activation Replace the interchangeable plastic retention element.

6. Resilient Anchor by Dr Biaggi. CM

Height 3.4 mm
Application The same as that described for Compact.
Activation Replace the split ring in the matrix.

7. Dalbo-B Spherical Anchor. CM

Height 4 mm
Application The same as that described for Compact.
Activation Using a special activating tool.

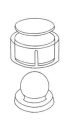

8. Shiner 'SR' Magnet System. Preat Corporation

Application Retention only of overdentures for root and implant abutments. The denture base, other abutments and root-faced attachments provide the stability.

9. Ceka Axial

Application To retain removable partial dentures or overdentures. To make this attachment resilient, the two space maintainers supplied must be used.
Activation Spread the segments of the patrix with an activating tool.

Bars

The bar, being the patrix, is attached to retainers while the matrix sleeve or clips/riders are processed into the denture. They are used to retain overdentures or removable partial dentures. The bar is usually soldered to two or more posts and diaphragms with enough space between them to allow the matrix sleeve or riders to be processed in the denture to give the necessary retention. They can also be used in conjunction with crowns and implants. They are either commercially or laboratory manufactured. Bars can be either rigid or resilient.

Rigid Bars

1. Rigid Dolder Bar. CM

Height 3.5 mm
Application Partial, hybrid and implant dentures. The Dolder bar cannot be bent to conform with the shape of the ridge or arch. A tapered arch may preclude its use.

Activation Bend both sides of the sleeve towards the centre with an activating tool.

2. Cast Laboratory Bar

This is constructed in the laboratory using a piece of plastic (1.25 mm thick) that will burn out in the furnace. The plastic is shaped to the ridge but cannot be shaped to the contour of the arch. The plastic is attached to the wax patterns, invested and cast. After casting, the bar is milled (see Chapter 6) and the retention supplemented by an auxillary attachment such as the Mini-Presso-Matic, Presso-Matic or Ipsoclip.

Resilient Bars

1. Ackermann Bar and Clip. MP

There are two types of Ackermann bar: one is round and the other egg shaped. The round bar is most frequently used as it can be bent more easily to follow

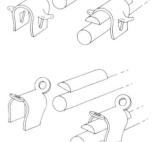

the contour of the ridge and arch. This allows more space for the clips, of which there are two types. One has lateral retention tags and should be used when there is reduced occlusal space. The other has the retention tags on the top of the clip. A brass half-round wire space maintainer is supplied and this is placed in the top of the clip prior to processing the prosthesis. When the processing cycle is complete, the spacer is removed, leaving a relieving space between the top of the bar and the undersurface of the clip.

Application Partial dentures, overdentures and implant dentures. The round bar can be shaped to follow the alveolar ridge.

Activation Bend both sides of the clip towards the centre with an instrument.

2. Round Bar with Rider. CM

Application and Activation The same as that described for Ackermann Bar and Clip.

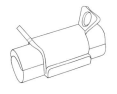

3. Dolder Bar Joint. CM

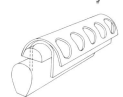

Application Partial dentures, overdentures, and implant dentures. Cannot be shaped to the alveolar ridge.

Activation Bend both sides of the sleeve towards the centre with an activating tool.

4. Preci-Horix

Application The same as that described

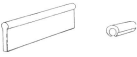

for Ackermann Bar and Clip. A plastic burn-out bar or metal bar is connected to the retainers; removable plastic riders in the prosthesis provide retention.

Activation Replace old riders with new.

Auxiliary Attachments

This group of attachments covers a wide range of applications. They can be used to: (a) allow contingency planning which will enable the clinician to remove the prosthesis for repair or conversion; (b) overcome alignment problems which arise when abutments converge, making it impossible to prepare them so that they can be mutually withdrawable when constructing fixed partial dentures; (c) replace the loss of soft tissue in anterior fixed partial dentures. Supplements retention on bars and telescopic crowns.

1. Mini-Presso-Matic. MP

Application To retain fixed operator-removable partial dentures that can be transformed into a patient-removable partial denture by replacing the screw bolt and hollow screw with the spring-loaded retention stud.

Activation Replace the spring and plunger.

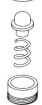

2. Presso-Matic. MP

Application To supplement the retention on milled laboratory-made bars and telescopic crowns used to retain removable partial dentures and overdentures.

Activation Replace the plastic cushion and plunger.

3. Ipsoclip. CM

Application The same as that described for Mini-Presso-Matic. Access to the spring and retention stud can be from either the front or the back of the attachment.

Activation Replace the coil spring and retention stud.

4. Epiloc/Gaussen Retentive Element. CM

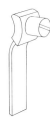

Application To retain the patient-removable anterior flange in fixed partial dentures.

5. Stabilizer and Ceccato Interlock. CM

Application Used as part of the bracing

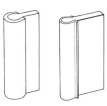

support to protect a slide attachment retaining a removable partial denture and as a substitute for guiding grooves.

6. Screw and Tube. CM and MP

Application To overcome minor and major withdrawal problems where abutments cannot be paralleled and to provide contingency planning for long-span fixed partial dentures and full-arch restorations when used in conjunction with inner thimble crowns. When the final treatment plan has been established, it is advisable to consult the manufacturer's manual when deciding on the appropriate alloy to use for the attachments.

Suppliers of Precision Attachments

1. MP. Metalor
Metaux Precieux SA Metalor
Dental Division
Av. du Vignoble
CH-2000 Nuechatel
Switzerland

2. CM. Cendres & Metaux SA
Bozingenstrasse 122
CH-2501 Biel-Bienne
Switzerland

3. Ceka. Ceka NV
Ceka Center
Noorderlaan 79, bus 1
B-2030 Antwerpen
Belgium

4. Preci-Horix. Alphadent NV
Ceka Center
Noorderlaan 79, bus 2
B-2030 Antwerpen
Belgium

5. APM-Sterngold
23 Frank Mossberg Drive
PO Box 2967
Attleboro MA 02703-0967
USA

6. Preat. Preat Corporation
1120 Seventh Avenue
San Mateo, CA 94402
USA
800-232-7732
(Ex. CA) 415-342-5700

Bibliography

Ackermann H. Ein neuer halter für stegpros-thesen. Schweiz Mschr Zahnheilk 67: 1013.

Amsterdam M. Periodontal prosthesis: Twenty-five years in retrospect. Alpha Omegan 67: 9-52, 1974.

Barker RM; Harrison A; Ralph JP. Overdentures in General Dental Practice. London: British Dental Journal, 1993.

Bennett AG. The vertical half-cap or bridge-work anchorage. Cosmos Dent 46: 367-369, 1904.

Brånemark P-I; Zarb GA; Albrektsson T. Tissue-Integrated Prostheses. Chicago: Quintessence Publishing Co, 1985.

Brewer AA; Morrow RM. Overdentures. 2nd Edition. Saint Louis: CV Mosby, 1980.

Burch JG. The dynamic mandibular arch width. In: Lurdeen HC; Gibbs CH (eds). Advances in Occlusion 81-87. Boston: John Wright PSG Inc, 1982.

Calclarone CV. Attachments for partial dentures without clasps. J Prosthet Dent 7: 206, 1957.

Carr CM. Anchored adjustable dentures. Cosmos Dent 40: 219, 1898.

Davis RK; Renner RD; Antos EW; Schlissel ER; Baer PN. Two year longitudinal study of periodontal health status of overdenture patients. J Prosthet Dent 45, 4: 358-363, 1981.

Dawson PE. Evaluation, Diagnosis and Treatment of Occlusal Problems. St Louis: CV Mosby, 1974.

Fossume FL. Removable and stationary bridges. Cosmos Dent 48: 859-860, 1906.

Ganne J; Astrad P; Ahten K; Borg K; Olsson M. Implants in partially edentulous patients: A longitudinal study of bridges supported by both implants and natural teeth. Clinical Oral Implant Res 3: 49-56, 1992.

Goslee HJ. Removable bridgework. Items Interest Dent 34: 731, 1912.

Grosser D. The dynamics of internal precision attachments. J Prosthet Dent 3: 393, 1953.

Guargiulo A; Wentz F; Orban B. Dimensions and relation of the dento-gingival junction. J Periodontal 32: 261-267, 1961.

Hobkirk JA; Schwab J. Mandibular deformation in subjects with osseointegrated implants. Int J Oral Maxillofac Implants 6: 319-328, 1991.

Hobo S; Ichida E; Goresia LT. Osseointegration and Occlusal Rehabilitation. Chicago: Quintessence Publishing Co, 1990.

Hollenback EA; Oaks S. Role of precision attachments in partial denture prosthesis. J Am Dent Ass 41: 173, 1950.

Jempt T; Book K; Linden B; Unde G. Failures and complications in 92 consecutively inserted overdentures supported by Brånemark implants in severely resorbed edentulous maxillae: A study from prosthetic treatment to first annual check-up. Int J Oral Maxillofac Implants 7: 162-167, 1992.

Jenkins WG. Bar anchorage systems for contingency planning. Independent Dentistry. Vol 1, No 2, May 1996.

Johns RB. Overdenture treatment with the Brånemark implant. In: Albrektsson T; Zarb GA (eds). The Brånemark Osseointegrated Implant 215-220. Chicago: Quintessence Publishing Co, 1989.

Jumber JF. Atlas of Overdentures and Attachments. 1st Edition. Chicago: Quintessence Publishing Co, 1981.

Kois JC. Altering gingival levels. The restorative connection. Part 1: Biologic variables. J Esthet Dent 6(1): 3-9, 1994.

Langer B; Sullivan DY. Osseointegration: Its impact on the inter-relationship of periodontics and restorative dentistry: Part II. Int J Periodont Rest Dent 9: 165-183, 1989.

Lee, JH. A new design of removable partial dentures. Practit Dent 14: 284, 1963.

Lee, JH. Sectional and partial metal dentures incorporating an internal locking bolt. J Prosthet Dent 13: 1067, 1963.

Lekholm U. Clinical procedures for treatment with osseointegrated dental implants. J Prosthet Dent 50: 116-120, 1983.

Lindquist LW; Rockler B; Carlsson GE. Bone resorption around fixtures in edentulous patients treated with mandibular fixed tissue-integrated prostheses. J Prosthet Dent 59: 50-63, 1988.

Miller CJ. Intracoronal attachments for removable partial dentures. Clin N Amer Dent 779, 1963.

Morison ML. Internal precision attachment retainers for partial dentures. J Am Dent Ass 64: 209, 1962.

Parel SM. The Smiline™ System. Dallas, Texas: Taylor Publishing Co.

Peeso FA. Crown and Bridgework for Students and Practitioners. Philadelphia: Lea & Febiger, 1916.

Preiskel HW. Overdentures Made Easy. London: Quintessence Publishing Co, 1996.

Preiskel HW. Precision Attachments in Prosthodontics, Overdentures and Telescopic Prostheses. Vol 2. Chicago: Quintessence Publishing Co, 1985.

Preiskel HW. Prefabricated attachments for complete overlay dentures. Brit Dent J 123: 161, 1967.

Preiskel HW. The use of internal attachments. Brit Dent J 121: 564, 1966.

Rangert B; Gurne J; Sullivan DY. Mechanical aspects of a Brånemark implant connected to a natural tooth: An in vitro study. Int J Oral Maxillofac Implants 6: 177-185, 1991.

Rangert B; Jemt T Jörneus L. Forces and movements on Brånemark implants. Int J Oral Maxillofac Implants. Vol 4, No 3, 1989.

Rieder CE. Copings on tooth and implant abutments for superstructure prostheses. Int J Periodont Rest Dent 10: 437-453, 1990.

Schuyler CH. An analysis of the use and relative value of precision attachment and the clasp in partial denture planning. J Prosthet Dent 3: 711, 1953.

Schweitzer JM; Schweitzer RD; Schweitzer J. The telescoped complete denture: A research report at the clinical level. J Prosthet Dent 26: 357-372, 1971.

Shillinbury HT; Hobo S; Whitsett LD. Fundamentals of Fixed Prosthodontics. Chicago: Quintessence Publishing Co, 1978.

Steiger A; Boitel R. Precision Work for Partial Dentures. Zurich: Stebo, 1959.

Tallgren A. The continuing reduction of the residual alveolar ridges in complete denture wearers: A mixed longitudinal study covering 25 years. J Prosthet Dent 27: 120-132, 1972.

The EsthetiCone: An abutment alternative for esthetic implant restorations. J Esthet Dent Update. Vol 2, No 2, April 1991.

van Steenberghe D et al. The applicability of osseointegrated oral implants in the rehabilitation of partial edentulism: A prospective multicenter study on 558 fixtures. Int J Oral Maxillofac Implants 5(3): 272-281, 1990.

Yalisove IL. Crown and sleeve-coping retainers for removable partial prostheses. J Prosthet Dent 26: 357-372, 1971.